Culture and Psychotherapy

A Guide to
Clinical Practice

Culture and Psychotherapy

A Guide to Clinical Practice

Edited by

Wen-Shing Tseng, M.D.
Jon Streltzer, M.D.

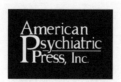

American Psychiatric Press, Inc.

Washington, DC
London, England

Copyright © 2001 American Psychiatric Press, Inc.
ALL RIGHTS RESERVED
Manufactured in the United States of America on acid-free paper

04   03   02   01   4   3   2   1
First Edition

American Psychiatric Press, Inc.
1400 K Street, N.W.
Washington, DC 20005
www.appi.org

Library of Congress Cataloging-in-Publication Data
Culture and psychotherapy   :   a guide to clinical practice   /   edited by
    Wen-Shing Tseng, Jon Streltzer.—1st ed.
        p. ; cm.
    Includes bibliographical references and indexes.
    ISBN 0-88048-955-3 (alk. paper)
    1. Psychiatry, Transcultural. 2. Psychotherapy—Cross-cultural studies.
3. Cultural psychiatry. 4. Cross-cultural counseling. I. Tseng, Wen-Shing,
1935– . II. Streltzer, Jon.
    [DNLM: 1. Psychotherapy. 2. Cross-Cultural Comparison.
WM 420 C9678 2001]
RC455.4.E8 C836 2001
916.89′14—dc21

                                                                            00-061805

British Library Cataloguing in Publication Data
A CIP record is available from the British Library.

Contents

PART 5

Special Models of Therapy

PART 6

Integration and Conclusions

Contributors

Iqbal Ahmed, M.D.
Professor and Vice Chair, Department of Psychiatry, John A. Burns School of Medicine, University of Hawaii; Program Director, University of Hawaii Affiliated Residency Training Program, Honolulu

F. M. Baker, M.D., M.P.H., F.A.P.A.
Professor, Department of Psychiatry, University of Maryland School of Medicine; Medical Director, Lower Shore Clinic, Salisbury, Maryland

David M. Bernstein, M.D.
Clinical Associate Professor, Department of Psychiatry, John A. Burns School of Medicine, University of Hawaii, Honolulu

Howard C. Blue, M.D.
Assistant Clinical Professor of Psychiatry, Yale University; Director of Clinical Services, Division of Mental Hygiene, Yale University Health Services, New Haven, Connecticut

Alan A. Buffenstein, M.D.
Assistant Professor, Department of Psychiatry, John A. Burns School of Medicine, University of Hawaii, Honolulu

Jose M. Cañive, M.D.
Director, Clinical Psychiatry Research, Albuquerque Veterans Affairs Medical Center; Associate Professor of Psychiatry, University of New Mexico School of Medicine, Albuquerque, New Mexico

Barry S. Carlton, M.D.
Associate Professor, Department of Psychiatry, John A. Burns School of Medicine, University of Hawaii; Chief of Psychiatry, Queen's Medical Center, Honolulu

Diane T. Castillo, Ph.D.
Psychologist, Albuquerque Veterans Affairs Medical Center and University of New Mexico School of Medicine, Albuquerque, New Mexico

Richard J. Castillo, Ph.D.
Professor, Department of Psychology, University of Hawaii at West Oahu; Clinical Professor, Department of Psychiatry, John A. Burns School of Medicine, University of Hawaii, Honolulu

M. Fakhr El-Islam, F.R.C.P., F.R.C.Psych.
Emeritus Professor of Psychiatry, Cairo University, Cairo, Egypt; Former Secretary, Transcultural Psychiatry Section, World Psychiatric Association

Ezra E. H. Griffith, M.D.
Deputy Chairman for Clinical Affairs, Professor of Psychiatry and of African and African-American Studies, Department of Psychiatry, Yale University, New Haven, Connecticut

Jing Hsu, M.D.
Clinical Professor, Department of Psychiatry, John A. Burns School of Medicine, University of Hawaii; private practice of psychiatry, Honolulu, Hawaii

Louise Jilek-Aall, M.D., M.A., D.Trop.Med., F.R.C.P.(C)
Clinical Professor Emerita of Psychiatry, University of British Columbia, Vancouver, Canada

Wolfgang G. Jilek, M.D., M.Sc., M.A., F.R.C.P.(C)
Clinical Professor Emeritus of Psychiatry, University of British Columbia, Vancouver, Canada; Former Chairman, Transcultural Psychiatric Section, World Psychiatric Association

J. David Kinzie, M.D.

Professor, Department of Psychiatry, School of Medicine, Oregon Health Sciences University; Founder of Indochinese Psychiatric Program, Portland, Oregon

Leslie Ann Matsukawa, M.D.

Assistant Professor, Department of Psychiatry, John A. Burns School of Medicine, University of Hawaii, Honolulu

Danilo E. Ponce, M.D.

Professor, Division of Child and Adolescent Psychiatry, Department of Psychiatry, John A. Burns School of Medicine, University of Hawaii, Honolulu

Jon Streltzer, M.D.

Professor, Department of Psychiatry, John A. Burns School of Medicine, University of Hawaii, Honolulu

Junji Takeshita, M.D.

Associate Professor, Department of Psychiatry, John A. Burns School of Medicine, University of Hawaii, Honolulu

Wen-Shing Tseng, M.D.

Professor, Department of Psychiatry, John A. Burns School of Medicine, University of Hawaii, Honolulu; Guest Professor, Institute of Mental Health, Beijing University, Beijing, China; and Honorable Advisor, Transcultural Psychiatry Section, World Psychiatric Association

Vicente B. Tuason, M.D.

Professor and Vice Chair of Psychiatry, University of New Mexico School of Medicine, Albuquerque, New Mexico

Preface

Modern societies consist of multiple ethnicities and are culturally heterogeneous. Mental health professionals inevitably find themselves treating people of widely varying backgrounds. Despite general recognition that culture influences psychopathology and also has profound implications for the practice of psychotherapy, only a handful of publications have specifically focused on culture and psychotherapy. This book addresses this need.

After publishing a book focusing on *assessment* of psychopathology (*Culture and Psychopathology: A Guide to Clinical Assessment,* Brunner/Mazel, 1997), the editors moved on to the present project, namely, the cultural aspects of *psychotherapy.* Much of the knowledge and case material in this book are based on clinical experiences and fieldwork with patients of diverse ethnic-cultural groups from several parts of the world, including the multiethnic society of Hawaii, the mainland United States, Canada, the Mideast, and India.

The contributors to this book are faculty members of the Cultural Psychiatry Study Group at the Department of Psychiatry, University of Hawaii School of Medicine, as well as many nationally and internationally known experts, some of whom have worked closely with the editors in the field of cultural psychiatry for many decades. The contents of the book have been carefully planned, organized, and edited in close collaboration with the chapter authors.

The book is subdivided into six parts. The first part serves as an introduction and overview of culture and psychotherapy. The second part comprises chapters in which the authors present and discuss the psychotherapy in a variety of cases with distinctive cultural issues and overtones. The third part addresses several specific issues in psychotherapy, such as cultural aspects of the therapist-patient relationship, and the giving and receiving of medication in the process of therapy. The fourth part focuses on cultural considerations in therapy for special populations, including adolescents, ethnic minority elderly, and some ethnic groups in the United States, including African American persons, Hispanic persons, and Southeast Asian refugees. The fifth part consists of chapters devoted to the interplay of cultural issues with certain specific models of therapy, including marital therapy for intercultural couples and group therapy with multiethnic members. The concluding sixth part is an integration and summary of the main themes of the book.

In contrast to many books on culture and mental health issues, this book does not primarily use specific ethnic groups as bases from which to elaborate on how to provide therapy for those particular ethnic groups, although this is done for certain prominent groups in Chapters 10–12. The intention is to focus on culture rather than ethnicity. Overall, however, the liberal use of case material allows examination of therapy situations involving a variety of ethnic groups encountered in North America, including Asian American, Native American, African American, Hispanic American, Polynesian American, and European American. Cases from the Mideast (Chapter 3) and India (Chapter 7) are included to illustrate the wide diversity of cultures. There has been no intention to include all ethnic groups, nor to emphasize any particular group. The cases are presented as tools to illustrate approaches to cultural issues in the treatment of patients and how culturally relevant psychotherapy must fit the ethnic-cultural background of each individual case in a unique manner. The message is that principles of transcultural psychotherapy may be applied no matter what the ethnic-cultural background of the patient.

The book is designed for use by psychiatrists, psychologists, residents-in-training, and related mental health workers. It should also be particularly useful in the teaching of culture and mental health. The book is primarily clinically oriented and is intended to be of value in the actual practice of psychotherapy. Literature is reviewed, general concepts are elaborated, numerous cultural issues that can influence psychotherapy are specified, and recommendations are made for clinical practice. In illustrating important issues, chapters frequently refer to actual cases that are reflective of clinical reality. Cases are chosen for their cultural interest, and the discussions of these cases always emphasize cultural concerns in psychotherapy, avoiding straying into general aspects of psychotherapy. Theoretical discussions of schools of psychotherapy are minimized in preference to a practical approach that stresses working with the cultural issues that may arise in any psychotherapy. For the sake of uniformity, the case material refers to the therapists in the third person, although most of the therapists were the chapter authors themselves. The patients' names and minor details have been changed to protect confidentiality.

We acknowledge the invaluable assistance of several people, whose contributions to the book were critical in bringing it to fruition. We thank Anne Taylor and Carole Kleve for their help with typing and production of chapter manuscripts, and Kathy Luter Reimers for her marvelous English editing, enhancing the readability and uniformity of the various chapters.

Wen-Shing Tseng, M.D.
Jon Streltzer, M.D.

PART 1

Introduction

CHAPTER 1

Culture and Psychotherapy: An Overview

Wen-Shing Tseng, M.D.

Prelude: Challenge for Clinicians

Contemporary mental health practitioners widely recognize the importance of cultural issues in psychotherapy. Knowledge of cultural factors and skill in dealing with them within the psychotherapeutic process are often necessary for a successful treatment outcome. The conduct of culturally appropriate and relevant psychotherapy can be quite challenging, however, particularly since cultural issues are often mystifying, misinterpreted, or even unrecognized.

Imagine, for example, doing psychotherapy with a Hispanic woman who presented problems of "losing her soul," or a Native American woman who could not escape her "spirit song," or an Irish patient who was concerned that he had done something not approved by his Catholic church. Dealing with psychological matters that involve supernatural or religion is an area that tends to be neglected in modern therapy, yet it is essential when treating patients from various cultural backgrounds who are oriented to supernatural beliefs.

In psychotherapy, what kind of professionally and culturally appropriate relationship should one build with a Japanese patient who was raised to respect authority figures and will not acknowledge feelings or opinions that he thinks will displease the therapist? To what extent, and in what way, should one encourage a Mexican patient to express his inner feelings and opinions to other members in a group session, when he culturally was taught *not* to reveal his intrapsychic thinking and negative feelings to others, particularly strangers?

When treating delayed grief reactions in a Vietnamese woman, a Samoan mother, or an African American woman, what kind of cultural considerations are necessary to help each patient resolve the trauma of loss? What differences in therapeutic strategies might be necessary for these patients of different cultural backgrounds? How might one understand, tolerate, and intervene in a culturally relevant way for a patient from mainland China or a Jewish patient from New York to resolve culturally accepted but clinically problematic dependency needs?

How would one conduct treatment with an underprivileged Native American adolescent as opposed to a socioeconomically affluent Caucasian adolescent? What determines the choice between individual psychotherapy or a group-oriented, action-based socio-occupational program to enhance ethnic identification? Should families be more involved in the therapy of Italian or Latino patients because of cultural values favoring the family system? Would one choose to conduct a more structured or more expressive family therapy for Scottish or Russian families? Would this depend on how they culturally stress the cohesiveness of family relationships?

These are questions that need to be considered and answered when conducting psychotherapy. They present challenges that modern therapists must confront daily in clinical practice in our increasingly multiethnic and culturally metropolitan society.

Clarifying the Concept of Culture

The term *culture* (*kultur* in German) was originally used in the late 18th century to refer to the achievements of civilization. However, the modern anthropological concept of culture was developed by a German scholar, Johann Gottfried von Herder, who advocated the idea that human beings had created a multitude of societies, each with its own version of human excellence (Prince et al. 1998). Following this conceptualization, scholars of anthropology redefined culture in various ways. The most commonly used definition is that of Kroeber and Kluckhohn (1952):

> Culture consists of patterns, explicit and implicit, of and for behavior acquired and transmitted by symbols, constituting the distinctive achievement of human groups, including their embodiments in artifacts; the essential core of culture consists of traditional ideas and especially their attached values; culture systems may, on the one hand, be considered as products of action, on the other as conditioning elements of further action. (p. 181)

Kottak (1999), a cultural anthropologist, delineated specific characteristics of culture: it is learned through a process of enculturation since childhood; it is transmitted through symbols, both verbal and nonverbal; and it is shared by members of groups. Culture is not a haphazard collection of customs and beliefs; it consists of integrated, patterned systems. People use culture creatively and actively. Culture can be adaptive and maladaptive.

The term culture needs to be distinguished from the terms *race, ethnicity,* and *minority,* which are often used incorrectly and interchangeably. To the layperson, race refers to a group of people that is characterized by certain physical features that distinguish it from other groups. Anthropologists use the term *geographic race* to refer a human population that inhabits a continental land mass or an island chain for a sufficiently long period and develops its own distinctive genetic composition and physical features, in contrast to other continental populations (Hoebel 1972, p. 232). African, Asian, Australian, Native American, European, (Eastern) Indian, and Polynesian are some of the major geographic races recognized around the world. Although races are assumed to have a biological basis, contemporary anthropologists now take the view that race is actually culturally perceived and socially constructed, and it is referred to as a "social race" (Kottak 1999, p. 41).

Ethnicity refers to the commonality of a social group whose members are distinguished from those of other groups by virtue of a common historical path; certain shared beliefs, values, habits, customs, and behavior norms; and a sense of group identity. Thus, culture refers to behavior patterns and value systems, while ethnicity refers to a group of people who share common cultural features (Tseng 1997).

Minority refers to a population group that is much smaller than the majority group in a society. Minority status may be related to race, ethnicity, or simply a sociohistorical path. Sometimes a minority group can be the most privileged—such as a colonizer of native people. More often, however, the minority is less privileged from political, economic, educational, and other perspectives and is frequently discriminated against psychologically or socially by the majority or the dominant group. As a result, the members of the minority group are vulnerable to conflict related to maintaining a strong minority identity versus assimilating into the majority culture.

Thus, theoretically, race, ethnicity, and minority have their own definitions and implications that should not be equated with culture. Culture should be reserved as a term and concept that refers to a set of beliefs, attitudes, and value systems that derive from the early stages of life through enculturation and become an internal mode of regulating behavior, action, and emotion. Thus, by definition, every individual, as a member of a group or a society, has his or her own cultural mode, regardless of his or her race, ethnicity, or minority/majority status.

Although by definition culture is transmitted from generation to generation, it is not entirely of a static nature. Culture changes continuously and dynamically through the generations in response to environmental demands. Thus, for example, immigrants of first, second, and third generations may have rather different subcultural systems that they observe and follow. Also, in relation to the size of the population, there can be many subcultural groups within a homogeneous society or within the specific groups in a multicultural society. Thus, in clinical practice, each individual needs to be assessed and the treatment managed in response to his or her own cultural system, without generalizing or stereotyping according to ethnicity or racial background.

Since culture is an abstract concept, relatively difficult to define and delineate, for the sake of convenience the term is often used in reference to ethnicity, race, or country. For instance, Jewish or Irish culture is addressed as ethnicity, African American culture as race, and Japanese or Russian culture by the names of the nations. However, caution is necessary in such use, because the unit of culture does not necessarily tie in precisely with the unit of ethnicity, race, or country. For example, China is composed of numerous minority groups, some of which have quite large populations, despite being labeled minority. The Uygur nationality, in the far west of China, has a population of nearly 6 million, and the Zhuang nationality, in the southwest, has a population of more than 13 million—larger than the population of many nations. "Chinese" culture, customarily referring to the cultural system of the majority Han nationals, does not reflect the Uygur or Zhuang cultural systems, which are distinctly different from that of the Han.

Furthermore, one needs to be aware that culture may be discussed at different levels. These include culture as an *ideal,* describing behavior that the culture strives for on the basis of cultural values; *actual* culture, describing behavior that is actually practiced and commonly observed; or *stereotype,* describing behavior that is often projected by others on the basis of partial observation and biased beliefs (Tseng 1997).

Lessons From the Study of Culture and Psychotherapy

The influence of culture on the theory and practice of psychotherapy has attracted the attention of psychiatrists, medical anthropologists, and mental health workers since the middle of the last century (Abel and Metraux 1974). Although "psychotherapy" can be defined as any psychological procedure that is aimed at relieving an individual's psychological suffering, such a definition can became problematic when it is discussed from a cultural standpoint (Prince 1980). For the purpose of cross-cultural elaboration, psychotherapy needs to be defined broadly as a special practice involving a designated healer (or therapist) and an identified client (or patient), with the particular purpose of solving a problem from which the client is suffering or promoting the client's mental health. The practice may take various forms, and the fundamental orientation may be supernatural, natural, biomedical, sociophilosophical, or psychological (Tseng 1999). The nature of psychotherapy has been examined from historical, universal, and cultural perspectives (Tseng and McDermott 1975), and the implications of psychotherapy in different cultures have been analyzed (Tseng and Hsu 1979). With regard to the practice and process of psychotherapy, the influence of culture has been explored from various directions (Tseng 1999) and is briefly reviewed here.

Indigenous Healing Practices

Traditional healing refers to nonorthodox therapeutic practices based on indigenous cultural traditions that operate outside official health care systems (Jilek 1994). Indigenous or folk healing involves various kind of practices, including religious healing, spirit mediumship (shamanism or a trance-based healing system), divination or various kinds of fortune-telling (including astrology or physiognomy), and the practice of meditation.

Reviewing various forms of folk therapy, Frank (1961) concluded that the core of their effectiveness lies in the therapist's ability to arouse hope by capitalizing on the patient's dependency on others. Comparing traditional and modern therapy, Torrey (1986) observed that both types of treatment have common therapeutic factors. The client's expectations of therapy and emotional arousal are usually enhanced by the therapeutic setting, and there is an emerging sense of learning and mastery. In both types of therapy, the therapist is able to decrease anxiety by identifying what is wrong with the client (naming effect), and the therapist usually possesses certain personality qualities that are admired by the client's culture.

Culturally Specific Psychotherapies

Although any form of psychotherapy is more or less under the influence of culture, some therapies are strongly colored by the philosophical concepts or value systems of the society in which the therapy was invented. Therefore, such therapy may be difficult to transplant to other cultures. Morita therapy, invented in Japan in the Meiji era; Rapid Integrated Therapy, fashionable in China during the period of the Great Leap Forward movement in the 1960s; and est (Erhard Seminars Training), popular in the United States during the 1970s, are examples. Comparison of culturally specific therapies to mainstream modes of therapy can provide a useful means of examining the cultural aspects of therapy (Lebra 1976).

Culturally specific therapies commonly use culturally consonant social ideologies to stimulate therapeutic improvement. Examples include fostering the Zen philosophical attitude of "accepting things as they are" for neurotic patients in Morita therapy; regaining self-confidence and enhancing social acceptance to meet politically demanded rapid recovery in Rapid Integrated Therapy; or expanding the experience of aliveness and full self-expression in est. Such therapies are often applicable only to particular sociocultural environments in given eras (Tseng 1999).

Cultural Elements in Mainstream Therapies

Even though many modes of therapy in the contemporary mainstream, such as analytically oriented therapy or cognitive-behavioral therapy, have been considered to have universally applicable techniques and theories, close examination reveals that no psychological therapy is immune from cultural influence. For instance, Meadow and Vetter (1959) pointed out how the Judaic culture's value system influenced the Freudian theory of psychotherapy. Judaism maintains that the ultimate goal of human happiness is attainable in the real world and that any unhappiness in real life needs to be fixed—which is the basic attitude reflected in psychoanalytic theory and is the purpose of therapy. To the Talmudic scholar, a word is presumed to possess a special hidden significance in addition to its direct meaning—similar to the view maintained by psychoanalysis of the meaning of words.

Interpersonal therapies, including family and group therapies, whose main focus is working on interpersonal relations, are very much in need of cultural adjustment. They need to consider how interpersonal interactions, relationships, or group dynamics differ among people in different cultural systems.

Societal Influence on Psychotherapy

Historically, the development of psychotherapy has been influenced not only by professional knowledge and theories but also by the sociocultural environment. Psychoanalysis never flourished in old Vienna, where it originated, because Vienna had a conservative society with many other ways of providing mental tranquillity for people and did not respond enthusiastically to this new method of treatment. However, psychotherapy became popular in the new world of America, where making changes in society and creating one's own life were valued in the country's pioneer atmosphere (Schick 1973). The acceptance of psychotherapy has also been obstructed by political ideology, as in Germany during the Nazi era, in Russia during Stalin's time, and in China during the Cultural Revolution.

The practice of psychotherapy is strongly influenced by the socioeconomic-medical system. In Scandinavian societies, where medical practice is heavily oriented toward their socialist systems, emphasis is placed on community-related health programs rather than individually focused psychotherapy (Kelman 1964). In many countries, such as Japan or China, "talking therapy" is not valued by people as much as ordinary medical treatment that uses medication or surgical procedures, and medical insurance may insufficiently reward a psychotherapist. In such societies, psychotherapy is not likely to be prevalent. In the United States, the fate of long-term psychotherapy is facing a severe challenge from changes in the medical care system, including the advent of managed care. These issues illustrate that the operation of psychotherapy is subject to many social factors beyond specific cultural influences.

Culturally Appropriate Care for Ethnic Groups and Minorities

Stimulated by the human rights movement, in the last three decades there has been a sharp increase in the awareness of and concern with the provision of culturally appropriate mental health services for minorities, particularly in the United States. These services include the provision of culturally relevant, responsive, and meaningful psychotherapy. Numerous publications have appeared that address the need for mental health care specific to various ethnic groups and minorities (Gaw 1982; McGoldrick et al. 1982; Tseng et al. 1974). Such books review basic cultural knowledge about particular ethnic/racial or minority groups, and they stimulate the awareness of cultural diversity among people in the same society (Comas-Diaz and Griffith

1988; Gaw 1993) or among ethnic/racial groups in different geographic regions around the world (Al-Issa 1995). Yet, such resource books may leave the reader with a stereotyped view of the particular ethnic or cultural group concerned. A clinician needs to know how to provide meaningful and effective therapy for *each* patient with *individualized* consideration consonant with the patient's individual cultural system.

Intercultural Psychotherapy

Intercultural psychotherapy refers to therapy that takes place between a therapist and patient of such remarkable differences that the cultural gap between them becomes a crucial issue in the process of therapy (Hsu and Tseng 1972). Associated with clinical experiences of working with patients in foreign societies, with persons in ethnic minority groups, and with increasing numbers of intercultural migrants from around the world, this subject has attracted a great deal of attention worldwide during recent decades.

There are numerous issues to contend with when doing intercultural psychotherapy. In addition to matters of transcultural communication and assessment, therapy is affected by the congruence and incongruence of cultural background between the therapist and patient, the possibility of racially biased beliefs on either side, the problem of ethnic or cultural identification with the therapist, and, in general, ethnic/cultural transference and countertransference (Hsu and Tseng 1972; Pedersen et al. 1989).

Culturally Relevant Psychotherapy for Each Patient

Thus far, most of the discussion of culture and psychotherapy has been about sociocultural factors that have a gross impact on the practice of psychotherapy as a system. Cultural issues often permeate the psychotherapeutic process in more subtle ways, however, which tend to be specific to the individual patient and related circumstances.

The experienced psychotherapist typically tailors the treatment to each patient's particular situation, depending on personal factors, the nature of the psychopathology, the stage of therapy, and so on. However, therapy can be most effective when another layer—the cultural dimension—is factored in. There is no special style or school of therapeutic practice for patients of divergent ethnic/cultural backgrounds. Rather, culturally relevant therapy requires the therapist to adjust, expand, or modify his or her understanding and method of treating each patient by considering the patient's ethnic and cultural background. To reach an appropriate level of cultural sensitivity and competence, the clinician needs to increase his or her cultural knowledge and expand or alter the treatment accordingly, and this needs to be done on a case-by-case basis.

Culturally relevant psychotherapy involves the management of cultural influences at multiple levels, including understanding how culture enhances the meaning of the patient's life history, clarifies the nature of any stress that may be encountered, alters the coping patterns utilized, and influences the psychopathology present. It also involves comprehending the cultural components of the patient's illness and help-seeking behaviors, as well as the patient's expectations of the therapist. As for the process of therapy, determining culturally relevant ways to communicate, establishing the therapeutic relationship, and understanding personal and ethnic transference as well as countertransference are challenges for the therapist. He or she must also determine the most culturally suitable goals, models, and techniques of therapy, while constantly examining whether his or her choices in this regard reflect personal values or patient needs. There is no simple recipe for the therapist to follow in making these choices, but the principles involved apply to all patients, whether minority or majority, of whatever ethnic background. Each case requires individual, dynamic adjustment. This case-oriented, practical approach is the main focus of this book.

References

Abel TM, Metraux R: Culture and Psychotherapy. New Haven, CT, College and University Press, 1974

Al-Issa I (ed): Handbook of Culture and Mental Illness: An International Perspective. Madison, CT, International Universities Press, 1995

Comas-Dias L, Griffith EEH (eds): Clinical Guidelines in Cross-Cultural Mental Health. New York, Wiley, 1988

Frank JD: Persuasion and Healing: A Comparative Study of Psychotherapy. New York, Schocken Books, 1961, p 62

Gaw A (ed): Cross-Cultural Psychiatry. Boston, MA, John Wright, 1982

Gaw A (ed): Culture, Ethnicity, and Mental Illness. Washington, DC, American Psychiatric Press, 1993

Hoebel EA: Anthropology: The Study of Man. New York, McGraw-Hill, 1972

Hsu J, Tseng WS: Intercultural psychotherapy. Arch Gen Psychiatry 27:700–705, 1972

Jilek W: Traditional healing in the prevention and treatment of alcohol and drug abuse. Transcultural Psychiatric Research Review 31:219–258, 1994

Kelman H: Psychotherapy in Scandinavia—an American viewpoint. Int J Soc Psychiatry 10:64–72, 1964

Kottak CP: Mirror for Humanity: A Concise Introduction to Cultural Anthropology, 2nd Edition. Boston, MA, McGraw-Hill College, 1999

Kroeber AL, Kluckhohn C: Culture: A Critical Review of Concepts and Definition [Papers of the Peabody Museum of Archaeology and Ethnology, Vol 47, No 1]. Cambridge, MA, Harvard University, 1952

Lebra WP: Preface, in Culture-Bound Syndromes, Ethnopsychiatry, and Alternative Therapies. Edited by Lebra WP. Honolulu, University Press of Hawaii, 1976, pp vii–x

Meadow A, Vetter HJ: Freudian theory and the Judaic value system. Int J Soc Psychiatry 5:197–207, 1959

McGoldrick M, Pearce JK, Giordano J (eds): Ethnicity and Family Therapy. New York, Guilford, 1982

Pedersen PB, Dragusn JG, Lonner WJ, et al (eds): Counseling Across Cultures, 3rd Edition. Honolulu, University of Hawaii Press, 1989

Prince R: Variations in psychotherapeutic procedures, in Handbook of Cross-Cultural Psychology, Vol 6: Psychopathology. Edited by Triandis HC, Draguns JG. Boston, MA, Allyn & Bacon, 1980, pp 291–349

Prince RH, Okpaku SO, Merke L: Transcultural psychiatry: a note on origins and definitions, in Clinical Methods in Transcultural Psychiatry. Edited by Okpaku SO. Washington, DC, American Psychiatric Press, 1998, pp 3–17

Schick A: Psychotherapy in old Vienna and New York: cultural comparisons. Psychoanal Rev 60:111–126, 1973

Torrey EF: Witchdoctors and Psychiatrists: The Common Roots of Psychotherapy and Its Future. New York, Harper & Row, 1986, pp 73–74

Tseng WS: Overview: culture and psychopathology, in Culture and Psychopathology: A Guide to Clinical Assessment. Edited by Tseng WS, Streltzer J. New York, Brunner/Mazel, 1997, pp 1–27

Tseng WS: Culture and psychotherapy: review and suggested practical guidelines. Transcultural Psychiatry 36:131–179, 1999

Tseng WS, Hsu J: Culture and psychotherapy, in Perspectives on Cross-Cultural Psychology. Edited by Marsella AJ, Tharp RG, Ciboroski TJ. New York, Academic Press, 1979, pp 333–345

Tseng WS, McDermott JF Jr: Psychotherapy: historical roots, universal elements, and cultural variations. Am J Psychiatry 132:378–384, 1975

Tseng WS, McDermott JF Jr, Maretzki TW: People and Cultures in Hawaii: An Introduction for Mental Health Workers. Honolulu, Transcultural Psychiatry Committee, Department of Psychiatry, University of Hawaii School of Medicine, 1974

PART 2

Case Presentations and Analysis

CHAPTER 2

The Man Who Became a Child in the Face of Death

Jon Streltzer, M.D.

Case Report

This case involves psychotherapy under somewhat nontraditional circumstances: the patient was treated in a general hospital while dying of terminal cancer. The therapy included collateral sessions with the wife as well as family therapy. Cultural issues were, for the most part, fairly subtle and involved differences in role perception between the dying man and his wife. Recognition of the cultural issues, however, was critical to solving the conflict in a manner acceptable to all. As the case is presented in this chapter, the thoughts of the treating psychiatrist are represented by the paragraphs in italics.

The Initial Presentation: A Dying Patient

An oncologist requested a psychiatric consultation for a hospitalized patient who was in the terminal stages of stomach cancer. The oncologist asked for

15

help in managing the patient's pain, and he also mentioned that the patient was unusually anxious about his condition.

Mr. Furukawa was a 47-year-old married man, the son of Japanese immigrants. He was a successful self-employed accountant, and he had one child, a 19-year-old daughter. The oncologist estimated that Mr. Furukawa had only a few weeks to live, and it was unlikely he would ever leave the hospital. The goal of medical treatment at this point was simply to keep the patient comfortable.

At the initial interview, the patient was seen in his hospital room, with his wife present. They were both quite cooperative with the psychiatrist. Mr. Furukawa was alert and fully oriented; there was no evidence of cognitive impairment. Mr. Furukawa had just received an injection of pain medication and was relatively comfortable, although he stated that pain was a significant problem much of the day. He was not sedated by the pain medication.

After discussing his problem with pain, Mr. Furukawa immediately volunteered that, through his own investigation, he had found a special type of vitamin therapy, which reportedly had a good success rate in curing cancer. He asked his wife to open a suitcase to show the psychiatrist the vials of medicine, which he had obtained in Japan. His oncologist did not know much about this treatment but was willing to let him take this medication, as long as he also accepted conventional medical care for his cancer. Mr. Furukawa had been taking these vitamin solutions for several months. It was obvious that his condition had deteriorated greatly during this period of time, but he expressed great optimism that the treatments could still work. He asked if the psychiatrist knew anything about these treatments or had any related information that might help cure his cancer.

The wife did not talk much during this initial interview. When the psychiatrist asked if this special Japanese treatment was commonplace in Japan, she spontaneously offered that other Japanese doctors did not recommend it or had not heard of it, but that patients came from all over to get it.

At the end of the first interview, the psychiatrist stated he would make some recommendations with regard to pain management and that he would be back to follow up.

This seemed to be a nice couple trying to cling to the hope that death could be avoided. The pain management would probably be routine. The case was likely to involve little more than providing support. It would not be difficult to satisfy the oncologist.

The psychiatrist recommended to the oncologist that the patient be given the long-acting analgesic methadone for pain in a slightly higher equivalent dose than that given in his previous regimen. The psychiatrist indicated he would follow the patient and his family for emotional support. The oncologist was very appreciative.

The Problem Surfaces

At the next visit, as a result of the changes in pain medication, the patient reported that he was feeling much more comfortable and yet was not overly sedated. In fact, he felt more optimistic in general, because he was feeling better. The psychiatrist took the opportunity to learn more about the patient's background and employment.

After the conclusion of the interview, the psychiatrist left the room, but the wife followed him out, wanting to talk to him alone. The wife, who, like her husband, appeared to be second-generation Japanese, told the Caucasian psychiatrist that it might not seem obvious, but her husband was actually having an extremely difficult time accepting his cancer. She noted that during the psychiatrist's interview, her husband seemed very rational, agreeable, and in a good mood, but this was only because, as a Japanese man, he needed to appear that way to his doctor.

The psychiatrist listened and then responded, "I'm very glad that you are letting me know about this so that I can be more sensitive toward your husband. I imagine this whole situation is very difficult for *you,* also." The wife then became tearful. For a moment she had difficulty responding but finally said, "Perhaps I am the one who needs your help more." Arrangements were then made for the wife to see the psychiatrist in his office in order to talk at more length about the situation.

The situation no longer seemed so clear. The wife was more distressed than the husband, and she insinuated that the psychiatrist does not fully grasp what is going on because of a "cultural gap" [see Tseng and Streltzer 1997]. Perhaps she just needed help in grieving, but perhaps there was more to it, and an exploration of cultural backgrounds would be in order.

Two days later, the psychiatrist met with Mrs. Furukawa. She immediately stated that she felt on the verge of a nervous breakdown. Her husband was being totally insensitive to her and expected her to wait on him hand and foot. He was obsessed with finding a cure for his cancer, and that was all he would talk about. He expressed no concern about his wife's and his daughter's lives or their futures. She knew he was dying, and she felt guilty for finding fault with him and was unable to discuss her feelings with him.

To make matters even worse, her husband's elder sister was showing up at the hospital every day. She was continuously babying the husband, increasing his dependency and demandingness. The sister had decided that a relative should be with her husband at all times and had worked out a rotation schedule, with family members signed up for different blocks of time. Mrs. Furukawa was relegated to being just another family member.

Mrs. Furukawa recalled that, when she married Mr. Furukawa, his sister had been against the marriage. Possibly this was because her family came from Okinawa, and Mr. Furukawa's family, particularly his sister, did not feel that she was the right kind of Japanese woman for him. As a result, Mrs. Furukawa and her sister-in-law had always had a cool relationship. Now, at this critical time, Mrs. Furukawa worried that her sister-in-law was trying to displace her as the most important woman in Mr. Furukawa's life. Mr. Furukawa seemed oblivious to this and even enjoyed all the attention from his sister. To Mrs. Furukawa, her husband was behaving like a spoiled child.

The psychiatrist explored the nature of the marital relationship. Mrs. Furukawa had very mixed feelings. Although Mr. Furukawa was an absolutely reliable and responsible husband and an excellent provider, he was difficult to communicate with, and Mrs. Furukawa would have liked to have received more affection and appreciation in the marriage. Mrs. Furukawa had come to accept her husband's personality, but it was clear that the daughter was affected by the lack of direct communication and attention from her father. Mrs. Furukawa also expressed concern that perhaps her husband shared his elder sister's belief that Mrs. Furukawa came from an inferior background, relegating her to an inferior role in the relationship.

The psychiatrist attempted to conclude the session with several therapeutic maneuvers. He tried to validate Mrs. Furukawa's feelings, praising her for bringing them out in the open. The psychiatrist also directly confronted Mrs. Furukawa's concern that her husband might perceive her to be culturally inferior. The psychiatrist pointed out that her husband had married her despite antagonistic feelings from his family, proving that he valued her for who she was as an individual. In addition, it was likely that it was characterologically difficult for her husband to express his true feelings or even to be fully aware of them. The psychiatrist stated that he doubted very much that Mr. Furukawa was happy with the current state of affairs. The psychiatrist indicated that he was going to talk to Mr. Furukawa and that he would like to arrange a session that included Mrs. Furukawa and the daughter, in order to deal with the important issues that had been raised. Mrs. Furukawa was doubtful that her husband would be able to communicate in any way other than the ineffectual manner that had always characterized his communication. She feared that bringing these things up might just make her feel worse. The psychiatrist responded that he would talk to Mr. Furukawa and then get back to her.

Mr. Furukawa's regression, denial, and insensitivity to his wife and daughter were consistent with culturally sanctioned behaviors. Despite this, there were numerous problems. The patient was not dying in a particularly dignified manner. He was unrealistically fighting his prognosis and ignoring important needs of his family. His wife was quite angry with him, and, with the situation as it was, she was likely to have strongly ambivalent feelings upon his death and a great deal of guilt. Furthermore, the relationship between the wife and the husband's family would most likely be permanently scarred, much more than it already had been.

The patient had an obsessive-compulsive personality style and was desperately seeking to maintain some kind of control over his inevitable downhill progression. The patient felt helpless with regard to his self-identity as a good provider for his family. His only solution was to somehow, miraculously, get better so he could return to work. Mr. Furukawa's thinking needed to be restructured so that he could still fulfill his cultural role of providing for his family. However, he would need to do this in a more emotional and spiritual sense rather than materially.

Confronting the Patient

The next day, the psychiatrist visited Mr. Furukawa and spoke to him alone. As usual, Mr. Furukawa began by talking about his special vitamins and asked if the psychiatrist had learned any more about them. After a few minutes of talk about these superficial and essentially irrelevant matters, the psychiatrist began to gently confront the patient. Instead of asking the patient about his own feelings, the psychiatrist asked Mr. Furukawa how he felt his wife and daughter were coping with the situation. At first the question puzzled Mr. Furukawa. The psychiatrist gently persisted in this line of inquiry, however, and the patient eventually decided that his wife and daughter must be having a difficult time. He became tearful. He worried that he was no good to them the way he was. He could not do anything for them. He could not go to work.

The patient's reaction was reassuring. He was opening up—revealing himself and confessing. The psychiatrist now had confidence that he could guide the patient in a therapeutic direction.

The psychiatrist pointed out to the patient that he had been a wonderful provider and, in fact, was extremely important to his family. The psychiatrist could assure Mr. Furukawa of this, because he had specifically been told this by Mrs. Furukawa. The psychiatrist informed Mr. Furukawa that it was not the loss of his ability to work and bring home money that concerned his family, but rather the loss of him as a person. Furthermore, for the rest of their lives, their memories of him would be determined, to a great extent, by how he related to them now. Mr. Furukawa agreed that he cared more for his family than his work. Indeed, they were his reason for living. He acknowledged his inability to express his caring and affection directly, but he assumed that his wife understood the way he felt. The psychiatrist stated that it was his impression that she did not really understand this, nor did his daughter. They were quite distressed about the way he had been behaving, which they interpreted as his not valuing their importance or recognizing their needs.

Mr. Furukawa did not know what he could do. He had never been able to communicate easily with his wife, and he was totally unable to communicate with his daughter. This was the big failure of his life, as far as he was concerned. The only thing he knew how to do was work hard and support his family. The more inadequate he felt with his wife and daughter, the more he devoted himself to his work.

The psychiatrist pointed out that Mr. Furukawa's family was not aware of his feelings. The patient seemed happy to let his sister take over and push his wife aside. Mr. Furukawa acknowledged that it looked that way, but it was not what he meant. He appreciated his sister's concern and enjoyed all the attention that she gave him, but he did not want to see his wife pushed aside.

Mr. Furukawa began to recognize the conflict between his wife and sister. He recalled that they had never related well to each other. He had always thought this was rather silly, and his response had been to ignore the issue from the beginning. That had worked satisfactorily because his sister had not been very involved with his life, until recently.

Mr. Furukawa asked the psychiatrist what he could do to fix the situation. The psychiatrist, without hesitation, told Mr. Furukawa to direct his elder sister not to oversee his care in the hospital, and, specifically, to clear any plans with his wife. Mr. Furukawa agreed to tell his sister not to schedule family members to stay with him all through the night, because he needed more time alone with his wife and daughter.

The psychiatrist also told Mr. Furukawa that he needed to talk to his wife and daughter, and to do so in a way that reassuring, heartwarming, and positive memories of him would live on within them. Mr. Furukawa indicated that this was exactly what he wanted to do, but he did not know how or if he was capable of it. The issue was discussed for a while, and Mr. Furukawa agreed to meet with his wife and daughter in the presence of the psychiatrist, who would help him express himself.

It was gratifying that the patient could come out of his self-absorption and let himself be guided toward a resolution of the family's distress. But would Mrs. Furukawa respond? It would be disastrous if she rejected her husband's overtures. This was a distinct possibility, because of the long-standing nature of her resentments, and because Mr. Furukawa was not likely to be very articulate in trying to make amends. An advance meeting with Mrs. Furukawa would be needed before risking a family session. She would need to be prepared for what was going to happen, to give her time to absorb the idea that things could still be different. Only if she responded would the family meeting be scheduled.

Preparing the Wife

The psychiatrist then met with Mrs. Furukawa. He stated that it was important that she and her daughter come to a family session, which the psychiatrist would arrange. It was his impression that her husband cared deeply for them and that he needed to tell them about it. Mrs. Furukawa responded with a flood of emotion. She did not think such a meeting would do any good; it would just upset her more. She did not trust her husband's sincerity. She described years of disappointment in the marriage, to the point that she had given up. She was just going through the motions. It did not matter so much for her, but it hurt her daughter terribly. Her daughter needed a father yet felt as if she had none. The psychiatrist allowed and facilitated Mrs. Furukawa's ventilation. Her feelings were entirely understandable; it must have been very difficult living with a husband who was so distant and unresponsive.

After a while, the psychiatrist gradually shifted the focus of the interview. He believed Mr. Furukawa was sincere in wanting to express his love and caring for his family. When the psychiatrist indicated that Mr. Furukawa was going to tell his sister to stop doing all she was doing, Mrs. Furukawa seemed less rigid in her objection to the possibility of communication. She agreed to the meeting and said she would arrange to have her daughter there also.

The Family Meeting

At the time of the meeting, Mr. Furukawa's condition was deteriorating, and he could no longer ambulate. In contrast to previous sessions, however, this time, when the psychiatrist entered the room, Mr. Furukawa did not immediately begin talking about his physical condition and potential treatments. His wife and daughter were also in the room. They were sitting in different corners, and there was an awkwardness and tension. They were waiting for the psychiatrist, and they needed him to begin the meeting.

The psychiatrist was anxious about the session. What if the wife blew up at her husband, and what if Mr. Furukawa ended up feeling more like a failure than ever? What would be the daughter's role? The psychiatrist hoped that the good relationships that he had developed separately with Mr. and Mrs. Furukawa would allow him to influence the interaction by promoting the positive side of each party's ambivalence.

The psychiatrist introduced himself to the daughter, whom he had not met previously. The psychiatrist immediately started the session by discussing its purpose. He thanked the daughter for being present. He told her that he had talked with her parents and it was his feeling that there were some misunderstandings about certain issues that everyone wanted to resolve. He stated that it was obvious to him that this was a very strong family, with deep feelings of caring for one another. The frustrations and misunderstandings were so troublesome precisely because the family had so much love and caring within it.

The psychiatrist then indicated that Mr. Furukawa had some important things to say to his family, even though it was very difficult for him to communicate directly, as this had never been his style. With this introduction, Mr. Furukawa began to tell his wife and his daughter how important they were to him and how much he loved them. He told them that it was to provide for them that he devoted himself to his work. At first he spoke haltingly and unclearly, but the psychiatrist forced him to clarify what he was saying.

Mrs. Furukawa responded that she had always felt ignored by her husband. He did not seem to recognize or care about her needs, which deeply hurt her. The psychiatrist pointed out that if she felt deeply hurt, she must have cared immensely about her husband's feelings and behavior toward her. The daughter joined in, saying she felt ignored and that her father did not seem to have any interest in what was going on in her life.

Mr. Furukawa responded with genuine emotion. He became tearful. He said he felt extremely inadequate. He cared deeply about what was going on with his daughter and was eager to know, but feared that if he asked direct questions, he would be intruding upon her. The daughter responded that she did not realize her father felt that way and that it was important for her to hear about his feelings. Mr. Furukawa and his daughter began talking to each other. She went to his bedside and hugged him, and they both cried.

Mrs. Furukawa was still sitting in her chair looking uncomfortable. The psychiatrist brought up the issue of Mr. Furukawa's sister. Mr. Furukawa acknowledged that he had been oblivious to what was going on. He agreed to talk to his sister and to tell her to stop making all the arrangements with his relatives. This turned out to be a critical step for his wife. She relaxed, her anger dissipated, and she began to relate to her husband in a caring and concerned way.

Mr. Furukawa followed through on his plan to talk to his sister. She was not happy and, after their conversation, spent relatively little time at the hospital. His wife and daughter were there as much as they could be, and they were always pleased to see the psychiatrist when he came to visit. Mr. Furukawa stopped talking about magical cures for his condition and accepted that he was rapidly deteriorating. The family members shared their grief, but they were prepared for his death. Two weeks after the family meeting, Mr. Furukawa died.

His wife came to see the psychiatrist twice as an outpatient after her husband's death. She expressed anxieties about carrying on without her husband. She was grieving appropriately.

Analysis and Discussion

Initial Presentation of the Case

Initially, this did not appear to be a psychotherapy case. The oncologist desired psychiatric consultation, ostensibly to help with pain management. It is likely, however, that the oncologist sensed unusual tensions in this situation that made this case different from other cases of dying patients. His vague impression that something was awry made him pleased that the psychiatrist got involved in the case beyond simple suggestions about pain medication.

At first, the psychiatrist expected the consultation to be limited in scope. The patient was dying, and he appeared to have an involved, supportive family. He seemed to be in significant denial regarding his condition, continuing to expect a cure from the special medicine from Japan. Denial is not necessarily bad in a medically ill patient; it can be a useful and effective defense mechanism (Streltzer 1983–1984). Indeed, the patient was convivial when first seen and did not appear at all depressed.

Cultural issues were obvious from the beginning, but they did not seem very important. The patient was a second-generation Japanese American. The search for a cure in Japan obviously had cultural significance. Perhaps, the patient believed that his best chance for cure included some sort of return to his roots, or, perhaps, it was simply the fact of having Japanese relatives that made it likely that he would hear about a special curative treatment in far-off Japan. Certainly, his background allowed him to be particularly hopeful and enthusiastic about a "Japanese" cure. The seeking out and be-

lieving in a magical cure in a hopeless situation is a common clinical phenomenon and appears to be fairly universal without any clearly known culture
specificity. When the patient requested the psychiatrist to help make this
cure work better, the psychiatrist expressed interest in the Japanese cure,
while honestly indicating that he did not know what it could do and that he
had never heard of it. Thus, the psychiatrist chose not to confront the patient's denial, but not to actively support it either.

Recognition of Cultural Issues

It did not take long for more complex and more significant issues to be revealed. Mr. Furukawa's expectations of himself and of his wife were at significant variance from those of Mrs. Furukawa. Mr. Furukawa was unaware
of this. Mrs. Furukawa was unable to communicate her distress to her dying
husband, and she was becoming increasingly overwhelmed and disturbed.
The cultural issues involved in this conflict were quite subtle but critical to
the problem.

   Mr. Furukawa had always assumed the role of provider for the family,
but not the manager of the family. This division of roles is entirely consistent
with contemporary Japanese culture. Furthermore, the work ethic remains
quite powerful among Japanese Americans, and it influences attitudes toward dying more than with other American ethnic groups (Kalish and Reynolds 1981). After developing a terminal disease, Mr. Furukawa could no
longer go to work, bring in money, and be the provider that maintained the
family's well being and stability. Unable to envision or enact a different kind
of role for himself, he became obsessed with finding a cure so that he could
return to his natural role as provider (as income producer). Thus, to him,
the harder he worked at finding a cure, the more he was fulfilling his proper
obligation to the family. It is probable that Mr. Furukawa was actually aware
of his prognosis and the extremely slim chance of finding a magical cure.
Nevertheless, he perceived it as his duty to his family to pursue that end.

   His wife was second-generation Okinawan. To some extent, she was
"liberated." At least, she believed in a broader role for women than that commonly found in traditional Japanese culture. She had her own full-time employment. She had never viewed her husband's role to be merely a reliable
provider for the family; she wanted him to play a more integral part in the
emotional life of the family. She was not liberated to the extent that she could
articulate her desires and confront her husband, however, and thus for many
years she had harbored resentments at her husband's passivity and emotional detachment.

This long-standing irritation erupted into a crisis for the wife when her husband's elder sister entered the scene. The elder sister took over and relegated the wife to a subordinate role in the care of the dying Mr. Furukawa. Mrs. Furukawa had always perceived that the elder sister looked down on her; their relationship had remained quite distant. The elder sister may not have approved of Mrs. Furukawa because of her Okinawan ancestry, which is considered inferior by some Japanese. It is also possible, however, that the sister was taking a role similar to the traditional Japanese mother, who remains very close to her eldest son and often dominates the daughter-in-law, treating her rather poorly. In Japanese culture, this may actually be expected by all parties, and the daughter-in-law who submits in a subservient and respectful manner to the domineering mother-in-law is much respected (the suffering daughter-in-law, of course, has her opportunity to reverse roles when her son marries) (Lebra 1984). Mr. Furukawa seemed to appreciate his sister's actions. He went along with them and was oblivious to his wife's discomfort.

Cultural Awareness Leads to a Solution

This case involved a "cultural gap" (Tseng and Streltzer 1997) between the clinician and the Furukawas. The psychiatrist was Caucasian, and in this particular case, it was probably advantageous that he was not Japanese. Being outside of that cultural background, he could see the issues framed clearly. Furthermore, the Furukawas would have been less likely to have role expectations for him. The wife may have actually been more comfortable talking to a non-Japanese male, believing he would be more able to listen to her concerns and less likely to think in the same manner that her husband did.

The psychiatrist chose to solve the problem by reformulating the situation in a manner culturally acceptable to all parties, and one that would fit Mr. Furukawa's individual dynamics. By redefining what being a provider for his family meant, the psychiatrist provided the opportunity for Mr. Furukawa to accept a new approach, and he was willing to communicate this to his family with the psychiatrist's help. Similarly, the psychiatrist reinterpreted Mr. Furukawa's motives to Mrs. Furukawa in a way that satisfied her needs. With all parties now open to resolution of their conflicts, the family meeting became the perfect venue for catharsis and forgiveness.

The psychiatrist purposefully did not contact or involve the sister in the therapy. Therapeutic resolution of the family conflicts required having Mr. Furukawa take control of the situation away from his sister and give it back to his wife. The sister had not played a significant role in the family previously, and to have involved the sister would have undermined the wife's position. Fortunately, Mr. Furukawa did not have a need for his wife to be subordinate to his sister. He had no difficulty communicating with his sister and changing that dynamic.

After the family therapy session, Mr. Furukawa was no longer concerned with the special medicine from Japan. He no longer seemed to be in denial and was accepting of his medical condition. His concerns remained with his family and building on the good relationship that had developed. In retrospect, what appeared to have been major denial had actually been Mr. Furukawa's attempt to fulfill his role within the family as he saw it.

In conclusion, we see that cultural issues subtly permeated the dynamics of Mr. and Mrs. Furukawa and the family as a whole. Cultural issues contributed to the root causes of the conflictual situation but also provided the opportunity for resolution.

References

Kalish RA, Reynolds D: Death and Ethnicity: A Psychocultural Study. Farmingdale, NY, Baywood Publishing Company, 1981, p 139

Lebra TS: Japanese Women: Constraint and Fulfillment. Honolulu, University of Hawaii Press, 1984

Streltzer J: Coping with transplant failure: grief vs. denial. Int J Psychiatry Med 13:97–106, 1983–1984

Tseng WS, Streltzer J: Integration and conclusions, in Culture and Psychopathology: A Guide to Clinical Assessment. Edited by Tseng WS, Streltzer J. New York, Brunner/Mazel, 1997, pp 241–251

CHAPTER 3

The Woman With
One Foot in the Past

M. Fakhr El-Islam, F.R.C.P., F.R.C.Psych.

Case Report

This case involves psychotherapy with an Arabian woman from a traditionally polygamous society. Her psychological conflicts were related to cultural
changes in her society, including the evolving social status of women.

The Setting

The setting of the case presented here was the Middle East. The patient was
seen at the only psychiatric clinic under the Ministry of Health of the state
of Qatar, in the capital, Doha. The clinic received patients referred by primary care doctors and nonpsychiatric specialists, as well as self-referred patients. Psychiatric examination and treatment, including psychotherapy,
were free of charge for both indigenous and expatriate members of the population, which totaled 400,000. Most of the medical practitioners in primary
and specialist care were expatriate Arabs, whose somatic orientation led

them to attribute all illness to bodily disease, without the interest or skill to look for psychosocial factors. The patients, the majority of whom presented with somatic symptoms, colluded with the somatic orientation of the doctors and expected somatic treatments. A "talking therapy" (i.e., psychotherapy) could not do much to alleviate the patients' suffering, and responsibility for their relief lay entirely with the doctors.

The psychotherapist has to introduce his role by discussing common examples of psychosomatic sequences of events (e.g., palpitations after fear experiences) and examples of Arabic psychosomatic figures of speech in order to communicate to the patient the possibility of alleviating his or her somatic suffering by modification or moderation of his or her psychological experiences. The therapist also has to demonstrate to the patient his understanding of the socioculturally shared system of values, beliefs, attributions, attitudes, and practice related to the illness. In particular, recognition of possible supernatural etiology could help the therapist to cross the doctor-patient cultural bridge.

The patient whose case is presented here was referred to the psychiatric outpatient clinic by a cardiologist at the end of a series of specialist examinations, locally and abroad. Therapy was conducted in Arabic, without any language barrier or interpretation. The therapist was an expatriate Arab, who had his training in both general psychiatry and psychotherapy in the United Kingdom, including training in individual, group, and family therapies.

Clinical Presentation

The patient, referred to as Maryam, a Qatari woman, aged 39, presented for psychiatric attention with a variety of somatic symptoms. This was a last resort, after repeated failure to find any basis for her symptoms. She still expected somatic treatment, albeit of a different kind, from the psychiatrist. Psychotherapy had to be conducted along unorthodox lines, including both supportive and dynamic techniques, with active participation of family members from time to time, in order to accommodate cultural beliefs and practices. The patient lived in a community that was undergoing rapid social change, which made it possible for her to look critically at her traditional upbringing. Conflict about traditional concepts of family relationships, idioms of expressions of distress, and codes of practice, as opposed to their modern counterparts, formed the core of psychotherapy for Maryam.

Maryam had an 8-year history of tightness in the chest, associated with left inframammary pain, and headache. Sometimes, she had difficulty in going to sleep, which she attributed to the pain. Her appetite was capricious, but she was rather overweight. Repeated physical investigation locally and in England, Germany, and France revealed no organic causes for her symptoms. (In Qatar, indigenous citizens, especially those from high-status tribes, can be treated abroad at government expense if they report failure to improve when treated locally. Treatment abroad, even for minor ailments, is a status symbol.)

After extensive medical consultation abroad, Maryam came to the conclusion that doctors had no experience with cases like hers, as all of them seemed to look for something they could never find. On direct questioning about her mood, she said the pains sometimes made her anxious and low spirited.

Maryam was brought up in a traditional Qatari extended family household, which included her parental grandparents, a divorced paternal aunt with her two children, and a stepmother with her three children, in addition to Maryam's biological mother and seven full siblings. The parents were first cousins. As the eldest of his male siblings, Maryam's father was traditionally and legally responsible for the livelihood of the extended family. Maryam was the second in birth order in her full sibship. However, as the eldest daughter, it had been her duty, since reaching puberty, to help her mother in household chores and in looking after her youngest siblings. At the age of 12, she was forced, according to the then-prevailing norm, to leave school and stay at home to participate actively in domestic duties, in order to learn housekeeping and nurturing maternal roles. Her parents came from wealthy families that belonged to high-status tribes, and this made Maryam very likely to be sought in an arranged marriage at an early age. The two wives of Maryam's father lived, at the same time, in separate parts of the same house.

Although Maryam had little school education, her youngest sister received a better education, as more favorable attitudes toward the education of females developed in the Qatari society at large. Maryam's stepsister, also called Maryam, had an infertile marriage and developed a variety of somatic symptoms, to which she and her family attributed the infertility.

The patient, Maryam, married by arrangement at the age of 15 and now had six children and two grandchildren. She felt physically run-down by the rapid succession of childbirths and resorted to the use of oral contraceptives *without* informing her husband. She hid this from her husband because it was his "right" in this culture to have as many children as he considered appropriate to his high status and wealth.

The patient's relationship to her children was full of warmth and healthy concern about providing them with a better education than her own. Although the daughters were doing better at school than the sons, Maryam's husband "persuaded" one daughter to discontinue her school education at the age of 15 years to marry a distant cousin. Maryam's symptoms started around that time.

Although Maryam had been brought up in an extended family household, by the time she got married, extended family households started to break up into nuclear family households. Maryam lived in a nuclear family household but continued to live in the extended family as a functional unit. Several nuclear families within the extended family, or within the tribe, continued to have frequent social contacts and to help mediate conflicts, arrange marriages, provide support in crises, consult on business and property, and secure jobs through nepotism.

The Beginning of Therapy

During the initial interview, Maryam resorted to repeated sighing to express her distress about her tight chest feelings. By taking deep inspirations, she assured herself that her chest could contain as much air as she thought it should. She was fidgety during the interview. Her apparently "poor" eye contact was within social norms, as females are not expected to look at strange men while talking to them. Maryam had no idea about the possible psychogenesis of her somatic symptoms. She did not think she had any emotional problems, and she felt that her family situation was fairly typical. The issue of individual differences in vulnerability to the usual and common stresses never occurred to Maryam.

The Doctor-Patient Relationship

After 8 years of treatment by physicians, Maryam expected yet another form of somatic treatment (e.g., medication by the psychiatrist). She showed surprise, and even resistance, when the psychiatrist asked her questions about her personal feelings that no other doctor had raised. She expressed the socially shared belief that it is body welfare that concerns doctors, whose expertise enables them to "remove" bodily symptoms. Explanation of the mind-body relationship in simple terms helped to clarify this area, making use of Arabic proverbs, which describe a noxious situation as pain in the head, a rejected situation as nauseating, and sadness as pain in the heart. The last proverb meant a great deal to Maryam, one of whose main complaints was pain in the region attributed to the heart.

Maryam, her husband, and her father asked the psychiatrist not to include the family/tribe name in his psychiatric records in order to not stigmatize them. The therapist assured them about confidentiality of his records and of his personal responsibility should there be any leakage of the name or any information from the records. Next, the family members wanted to know what goes on in therapy, and even to attend treatment sessions.

In this conservative community, and for this ultraconservative family, the presence of an adult female with a male stranger (e.g., a doctor) in a closed room was not easy to accept. Maryam's relatives maintained that the psychiatrist should be able to "administer" any treatment in their presence, or at least in the presence of a female nurse. Privacy of information given by Maryam was discussed with family members as the essence of therapy; she could talk about unpleasant feelings toward family members, which she had not expressed for 8 years. It was her decision whether to tell family members about herself and/or her treatment. The therapist affirmed, however, that therapy could involve family members in joint sessions in the future. Maryam then described how her access to foreign doctors in England, France, and Germany was marred by interpreters, who were often her own relatives, because this limited her freedom to describe how she felt about her symptoms. Moreover, she had the impression that interpreters gave the foreign doctor their own version, summary, or conclusion, rather than the full details of what she wished to communicate. She felt non-Arab doctors could not understand her worries anyway, because her worries involve native ways of interpreting symptoms and concern about them.

It was ultimately possible to persuade Maryam that talking about her feelings could help her understand them through the eyes of someone else (i.e., the therapist), work through them in order to resolve conflicts, and adjust better in her personal and family life. She was motivated to accept psychotherapy as a last resort after a long sequence of somatic treatment failures. However, she felt insecure without medication, which she thought prevented her from getting worse. The therapist did not object to concurrent drug therapy with anxiolytic antidepressants, for the time being.

Psychotherapy: Behind and Beyond the Somatization

At the beginning of psychotherapy, Maryam talked a great deal about her somatic symptoms and the drugs and physiotherapy she received for them. The therapist declined to comment on these and punctuated by probing her feelings and thoughts about herself and various family members. The therapist's probes and quiet ignoring of her somatic talk gave Maryam a subtle directive message, and she gradually produced more and more information about her feelings and, later on, her fantasies. These disclosures were consistently rewarded by encouraging comments, until finally she no longer discussed somatic symptoms.

The onset of symptoms 8 years earlier had coincided with the marriage of Maryam's eldest daughter, at the age of 15 years. The patient's identification with her daughter was clear, not only because they married at the same age but also because both would have preferred to continue their school education and both were wed to cousins. As she became able to identify and talk about these and other angry feelings, she took more interest in making decisions within her nuclear family, and expressed determination that her younger children would achieve greater self-actualization through education and even in careers. It was as if Maryam wanted to relive her childhood through her children, to make up for whatever she had missed.

After the therapist's success in defending the privacy of information given by Maryam against her husband's initial attempts to intrude in therapy, Maryam took over and became assertive in her relationship with her husband. She also stood up for her children's rights when her sons tried to overrule her daughters, and when the older children tried to subdue the younger children, according to traditional codes of relationships within the family. The husband did not like the change in Maryam. He noted that she had become cocky and angry, and he asked to see the therapist in order to discuss this "unwelcome" change. The therapist asked the husband to discuss his request with the patient and, after she agreed, arranged a joint session.

During this session, it was clear that the conflict centered around interparental differences in attitudes toward their children, with Maryam being more "liberal." She encouraged their age-appropriate self-management and independence in choice of friends, television programs, and time for doing homework on school subjects. The husband was informed by the therapist that Maryam's approach proved to work in many families, and he agreed to give it a chance. This prevented his sabotage of therapeutic changes in his wife. As another Arab man, the therapist was expected originally by Maryam to take the side of her husband, but since he did not, she felt more confident to continue her assertiveness with less angry expressions. She later taught her children to discuss their thoughts and feelings directly with their father, without her having to act as their advocate. This largely eliminated a lot of angry exchanges between the couple.

After Maryam's reliance on somatic communication in body language diminished in both psychotherapeutic and family relationships, the increased reliance on verbal communication led to the emergence of several themes centered around envy. Maryam talked about her secret envy of the education she assured for her children and of their future occupational opportunities. Similar feelings were expressed in relation to her younger sisters, who had had a better education. She regretted the time she had had to spend as an assistant to her mother in housekeeping and care for the youngest siblings, instead of enjoying her late childhood and early adolescence. She was encouraged to identify with the achievements of her children, and, in fact, she read some of their books. When she discussed her readings with the children, they told her she would have been more successful than themselves had she completed her school education. This boosted her ego.

Another theme of envy involved Maryam's sister, who had a childless marriage that led her husband to acquire a second wife, who produced children for him. Maryam thought the sister envied her for having six children of her own. Whenever her children had health or school problems, she wondered whether the envying "evil eyes" of her sister could be responsible. From a traditional religious healer, Maryam obtained amulets containing verses from the Koran (the holy book of Muslims), which the children had to carry around their arms. She also increased her prayers to God, to ward off the envying eyes.

By temporarily suspending her child-producing function through the use of oral contraceptives, Maryam thought she was threatening her own femininity as defined by her culture. She felt guilty about not informing her husband about this and about transgressing Islamic religious rules about contraception and procreation. The neutral position of Islam in relation to contraception was explained, and she accepted this clarification from the therapist as a Muslim and commented on his strongly Islamic name. When the therapist wondered what Maryam thought would happen if her husband found out she was using oral contraceptives, Maryam said she thought he would explode and look for a second wife. However, she broached the subject by asking her husband what he thought about contraception in general. During the following session, she let the therapist know that she had told her husband a "white lie"—that the therapist had instructed her to tell him about her use of contraceptives. In a subtle manner, the therapist had actually given her permission to tell her husband the truth.

Contrary to her fantasy, her husband took the news about Maryam's contraceptive use quietly and said he had suspected it. They agreed she would give up the use of contraceptives in the future if her husband thought she should have more children. Maryam then felt she was appreciated by her husband as a person, and not simply as a child producer. For the first time, she admitted that she used to have fears of going off to sleep, lest she should die as a sinner, since she used contraceptives, and go to hell. She also had fantasies of torture in her grave after death for the same reason. These symptoms disappeared after resolution of Maryam's conflicts about contraception.

The psychology of Maryam's sexual development came into focus next. As she approached menarche, her mother and other women in the extended family household had told her about men's sexual desire for women. The menarche, she was told, would change her from a child to a woman, and men could use devious and even violent methods to have sex with her. She understood that the less she had to do with men the better, and that she should be escorted by a brother or another male relative to protect her whenever she went outdoors. However, she felt guilty about thinking that men were physically attractive to her. She wondered why men did not have to cover their physical attractions with clothes, whereas women had to be covered almost totally by Islamic clothing (hijab). During her final year at school, Maryam entered into lengthy discussions with her classmates on this topic, but they could never find answers to their sexual conflict.

Maryam's husband instructed her to prevent their daughters (and not their sons) from watching television programs that showed unconventionally dressed women or that referred to love or sex, because these programs were thought to reflect loose morals in other Arab countries, from which they were imported. Maryam did not approve of this discrimination. She asked the daughters, who had their own sets in their rooms, not to inform their father or brothers about the programs they watched. However, she discussed some of the programs with them and talked to them about the need to fit into the norms of their family and community. The sons, on the other hand, were allowed to watch culturally disapproved sex videotapes, which they kept under lock and key in their rooms.

Maryam expressed some conflict about her two Filipino maids. The youngest son bonded strongly to the older maid, who had left her own children in her home country. This maid spoke no Arabic, and the son had had some delay in language development but caught up after going to school. Maryam also suspected that her husband found the younger maid physically attractive. As a sign of affluence, having two maids was thought to arouse the envy of Maryam's neighbors, also. She needed the maids to look after the huge house they lived in, but she did not like their inappropriate emotional involvement with the family members. During the period of psychotherapy, Maryam replaced the resident maids by part-time nonresident maids and restricted their duties to manual work in the house. Although she took pride in remaining her husband's only wife for more than 20 years, she thought this was a source of envy in the extended family network.

Polygamy is still the rule in Qatari society. A woman who remains the only wife of a high-status, wealthy husband like Maryam's for this length of time has to be regarded as an exceptional woman, to have fulfilled all her husband's sexual and pronatalist needs. When a husband acquires an additional wife, it is not unusual for an earlier wife to develop a resistant somatization, or to subdue the new wife, in order to maintain herself as the overall head of the household. In theory, wives have the right to be treated equally in the physical, emotional, and material components of married life. In practice, competition for the husband's attention is common. Such competition can be overt or covert, by proxy, through involvement of the children's needs for their father, such as for health reasons, when they have to be taken by him to doctors.

Throughout psychotherapy, the therapist encouraged Maryam to have access to the feelings and thoughts that lay behind and beyond the somatic symptoms. She learned to examine her feelings and take action to resolve conflict. She dealt with feelings of envy by others, and fantasized transgression of the religious code, by direct appeal to God through reading Koranic verses and praying. Involving family members in Maryam's case was essential not only to affirm her right to confidentiality of information but also to avoid their discouragement, or opposition, to her change from somatically to verbally expressing her feelings. The therapist never criticized her beliefs about envy as unproved or disprovable, nor did he describe her resort to traditional healers as irrational. Self-reliance was encouraged in adopting religiously acceptable autonomous (autoplastic) coping, instead of dependent (alloplastic) reliance on traditional religious healers for help.

Maryam's need for further psychotherapy was discussed next. The issue of termination of therapy did not come as a surprise to her, at a time when her somatic symptoms virtually disappeared without the use of psychotropic medication. She was encouraged to take pride in her autonomous problem-solving ability. She agreed to termination of therapy, with the therapist's assurance of continued availability of professional help whenever she felt the need for it.

Further Contact After Termination

After termination of her once-a-week psychotherapy for 3 months, Maryam contacted the therapist twice during the next 2 years. She sought help when her husband tried to force another daughter to marry a distant cousin. The daughter preferred to continue her university education. A family therapy session was arranged as a crisis intervention. In the presence of her parents, the daughter explained the incompatibility between her and the prospective groom, who was less urbanized and much less educated. During this family session, the discrepancy in attitude and style between Maryam's daughter and the groom chosen by her father was discussed by the therapist, who added that when young people (male or female) approve of a spouse, this makes them more responsible and more tolerant in marital relationships, as they work harder to maintain and cement the marriage. It transpired that the daughter was in love with a university graduate, who belonged to another high-status family, to whom she eventually became engaged, with parental approval. The crisis intervention session helped the daughter to confront her father and secure his approval of her choice of another prospective groom. The daughter achieved what Maryam would have liked to have achieved.

The second occasion on which Maryam contacted the therapist was when cans of beer were found in her eldest son's room. She thought this was not only a break of the time-honored religious prohibition of alcohol but also a sign of her son's addiction. She had fantasized about her husband's physical violence toward the son if he were informed about this. In another family session, it became clear that the son did not fulfill the medical criteria of dependence on alcohol or drugs. He was only trying alcohol as were other young men he knew. However, he realized the strength of his parents' objection to the use of alcohol and agreed to no longer bring any to the parental home. At Maryam's request, the therapist explained the health risks of alcohol consumption. The son, who showed no interest in school education beyond the eighth standard, planned to join the army and live independently. He preferred a modest career in the army to joining his father's prosperous business, where he expected he would be constantly under his father's control.

Through the process of therapy, Maryam had become a happier and more contented person. She not only lost her somatic and emotional suffering but also became better adjusted and more capable of conflict resolution.

Analysis and Discussion

Although Maryam's symptoms were common and global, the underlying cultural psychopathology was unique to her Arabian Gulf community. Conflict between time-honored traditional codes and liberal modern pursuits often leads to *interpersonal* strife between conservative and liberal individuals (e.g., intergenerational conflict) (El-Islam et al. 1986) and *interparental* (i.e., intercouple) conflict (El-Islam et al. 1988a). The conflict is also *intrapersonal* (i.e., in each individual), between recently acquired values and parental values that were internalized during childhood and maturation. Major areas of conflict include family relationships, type of marriage, and the role of women in society. Since the acquisition of oil wealth, access to modernity has been possible in affluent Arabian Gulf communities, through the information media, tourism in modernized countries, and the employment of large expatriate communities. The last-mentioned, whose members form almost half of the total population, bring with them not only their expertise but also their liberal attitudes and codes of living. As an indigenous Gulf Arab, Maryam had one foot insecurely placed in past traditions, which had not died, and the other foot insecurely placed in present conditions, which were not certain to survive.

In keeping with local traditions, Maryam's husband was only the material power and disciplinarian authority in the family. He spent most of his leisure time socializing with male friends and extended family members in the guest areas (*majliss*) of his house or their houses. All emotional input and care was Maryam's responsibility in the family. Large families, often with around 10 children per wife, are still common in this polygamous community. Although foreign maids were frequently employed in these families in the past, many home managers, like Maryam, no longer involve them in bringing up their children. This is not only because of the language barrier but also because of the maids' ambivalence about caring for other children, while abandoning their own in their home countries for the sake of better earnings in the affluent Gulf countries.

Arabian Gulf patients share the expectation that the doctor's job is to remove their symptoms and cure them without active participation on their part. Therefore, Maryam needed persuasion in order to accept the active role of exploring her own feelings during psychotherapy. Maryam presumed that, because her therapist came from a more liberal Arab country, he would empathically understand both Arabic cultural traditions and modern aspirations like hers. She expected less of a patient-doctor cultural gap (Tseng and Streltzer 1997) in this particular therapy than in therapy conducted by European doctors she had seen previously.

Maryam's husband asked to attend her therapy sessions because it was his culturally enforced duty to know everything about her, his wife. Moreover, the Islamic religious concept of unauthorized dyad (*khalwa ghair shari'ia*) condemns dyadic encounters between a woman and a strange man in a closed room on their own. The devil (*Shaitan*) is believed to intimate illicit sexual thoughts and feelings to them in such a situation. The therapist had to explain that meeting alone was a standard practice in psychotherapy and to assure the husband that the therapist never found any evidence for these types of thoughts or behaviors in his practice. Explanation of the professional nature and strict confidentiality of the relationship secured the husband's permission for his wife to start individual psychotherapy.

Maryam believed women should have multiple roles in society, whereas the local culture assigns to women the monorole of procreation and mothering. Women who fail to fulfill their traditional roles (e.g., Maryam's sister) are regarded as social failures. They often develop multiple somatic symptoms, which become culturally accepted excuses for their failure (El-Islam 1975). On the other hand, psychological symptoms, which express emotional disorder directly without somatization (such as excessive worries, fears, or low mood), are traditionally attributed to weakness of faith and call for religious help to strengthen the individual's faith (El-Islam 1982). Initially, Maryam obtained help from religious healers, but, as she became more self-confident, she obtained such help autonomously, through her personal religious practice. The Islamic religious code prides itself on denying any mediating role for the clergy between God and humans, who should call Him directly for help. This was used to motivate Maryam's religious autonomy during psychotherapy.

Maryam's conflict about contraceptive pills led to cognitive dissonance. The Arab community has been traditionally pronatalist during the pre-Islamic and Islamic eras. There is a socially shared misunderstanding that the Islamic religion prohibits contraception. Psychiatric symptoms associated with the use of oral contraceptives were found to be more common among women who believed that contraception was against the Islamic religion than among those who did not adopt such a belief (El-Islam et al. 1988b). Maryam's other conflict about contraception involved the cultural value of having a large number of children. It is not only a source of respect for women but also a source of pride for men, as a sign of virility, wealth, and social status.

Marriage of females at a young age is still traditionally approved. Girls from high-status families are likely to be sought in arranged marriage at younger ages. Maryam and her daughter were cases in point, when they married at age 15 years. Their school education was discontinued because it was not traditionally valued for females. Sons are expected to go further in education and are given more authority in the family than daughters. However, in Maryam's family, a son showed no interest in education, while a daughter joined the university. Among members of the indigenous Gulf community, females typically do better in school education than males, as if the former were trying to demonstrate that they are worthy of a nontraditional role in school education and subsequent careers.

Another conflict that unfolded in Maryam's case involved awareness of her sexual arousal by physical attraction toward men. During childhood and maturation, females are traditionally conditioned to deny sexual feelings. Maryam felt guilty about having feelings that should not be experienced by "good" girls. Repression of female sexuality is traditionally considered better than risking the development of uncontrollable sexual feelings that could end in disgraceful premarital pregnancy. Maryam was brought up to believe that it is natural only for men to have sexual feelings toward females, who are regarded as objects of their sexual gratification.

After establishment of the proper doctor-patient working relationship, Maryam was able to describe and examine her feelings in rich verbal detail. Her ability to describe her feelings does not support the notion that somatic symptoms and body-oriented presentation are common in developing countries because their languages are poor in verbal description of emotional experiences (Leff 1973).

Among the indigenous Gulf population, there is a socially shared belief that expatriate Arabs, including doctors, have loose moral codes. It is therefore advisable, during psychotherapy, to avoid or ignore themes of patients' cultural transference and to discourage, as well, their marked regression and dependence on the therapist. For persons who are not familiar with the analytically oriented therapeutic procedure, transference interpretations of patients' emotional experiences and expressions may be taken by the patients and/or their relatives as implicit invitations for personal, nonprofessional involvement. This could lead to premature termination of psychotherapy and even litigation.

Conclusion

The psychotherapy of Maryam provides several examples of the implications of culture in clinical psychiatry in Arabian Gulf communities (El-Islam 1998). Contributions to Maryam's symptoms were made by culturally shared beliefs about the monorole of women in procreation and mothering and religious sanctions against contraception. Intergenerational conflict and interparental conflict about modern versus traditional orientations precipitated professional help seeking for restoration of family harmony.

In Maryam's case, cultural issues substantially affected the patterns of presenting symptoms, the doctor-patient relationship, and expectations from therapy. Since the family is traditionally the main agent of social welfare, it had to be involved as a support resource during psychotherapy. However, a line had to be drawn between the therapist's welcome of such support and his rejection of the attempt of some family members to encroach on the privacy and confidentiality of individual psychotherapy by claiming a right to know about the patient (El-Islam 1994).

Maryam's case illustrates the need for the therapist to appreciate the patient's cultural influences and stresses, and the need of all medical practitioners to know how to elicit evidence of psychosociogenesis of a patient's somatic complaints. Recognition of cultural influences allows the therapist not only to use culture as a therapeutic resource but also to maintain a homeostatic balance in family relationships by refraining from both the total rejection of old cultural norms and the total acceptance of modern norms. It would have been counterproductive to encourage gross outstepping of the pace of cultural change in the society at large. By allowing formal access of women to university and to employment, society has moved from a monorole to a multirole for women, but taboos on women's sexual needs are still enforced. Family relationships tend to become more democratic, without encroaching on filial piety and respect for elders. Thus, adequate cultural understanding of the patient, and of the society at large, allows the therapist to carry out a culturally relevant and successful psychotherapy.

References

El-Islam MF: Culture-bound neuroses in Qatari women. Soc Psychiatry 10:25–29, 1975

El-Islam MF: Arabic cultural psychiatry. Transcultural Psychiatric Research Review 19:5–24, 1982

El-Islam MF: Collaboration with families: an alternative to mental health legislation. Care in Place 1:256–260, 1994

El-Islam MF: Clinical applications of cultural psychiatry in Arabian Gulf communities, in Clinical Methods in Transcultural Psychiatry. Edited by Okpaku SO. Washington, DC, American Psychiatric Press, 1998, pp 155–170

El-Islam MF, Abu-Dagga SI, Malasi TH, et al: Intergenerational conflict and psychiatric symptoms. Br J Psychiatry 149:300–306, 1986

El-Islam MF, Malasi TH, Abu-Dagga SI: Interparental differences in attitudes to cultural change in Kuwait. Soc Psychiatry Psychiatr Epidemiol 23:109–113, 1988a

El-Islam MF, Malasi TH, Abu-Dagga SI: Oral contraceptives, sociocultural beliefs and psychiatric symptoms. Soc Sci Med 27:941–945, 1988b

Leff JP: Culture and differentiation of emotional states. Br J Psychiatry 123:299–306, 1973

Tseng WS, Streltzer J: Integration and conclusions, in Culture and Psychopathology: A Guide to Clinical Assessment. Edited by Tseng WS, Streltzer J. New York, Brunner/Mazel, 1997, pp 241–252

CHAPTER 4

The Woman Who Could Not Escape Her Spirit Song

Louise Jilek-Aall, M.D., M.A.,
D.Trop.Med., F.R.C.P.(C)
Wolfgang G. Jilek, M.D., M.Sc.,
M.A., F.R.C.P.(C)

Case Report

This case involves a Salish Indian woman in whom the dilemma of seemingly opposed cultural demands engendered a serious intrapsychic conflict, which was resolved in the process of psychotherapy. As the case is presented in this chapter, observations on the case by the treating psychiatrist are represented by the paragraphs in italics.

Background

In the traditional culture of the Coast Salish Indians of the Pacific Northwest, the *spirit song* represents the power of the guardian spirit, a concept shared by many North American Indian peoples (Benedict 1923). In the past, guardian spirit power was acquired individually in an arduous spirit quest, extending over years, in forests and on seashores. To hear one's spirit song was a sign of "spirit sickness" through possession by the guardian spirit. In order for the individual not to succumb to this sickness, but rather to utilize the power conveyed by the guardian spirit to one's great benefit, initiation to the spirit dance ceremonial was called for.

After many decades of official suppression, the guardian spirit ceremonial of the Coast Salish in British Columbia and Washington State was revived in the 1960s, in the context of the general renaissance of indigenous North American cultures (Jilek 1978). Although in modern times the traditional individual spirit quest was no longer practicable, the few surviving shamanic ritualists of the Salish saw themselves confronted with the therapeutic needs of many native persons with severe psychosocial problems, who were not being effectively treated or rehabilitated in the established Western medical or correctional systems. The Salish ritualists therefore reinterpreted the traditional concept of spirit sickness as referring also to depressive symptoms due to experiences of anomie, cultural identity confusion, and relative deprivation ("anomic depression"; see Jilek 1974), sometimes associated with substance abuse and antisocial behavior.

This modern spirit sickness is seen by Salish Indian ritualists today as the result of imposed acculturation and exposure to the negative aspects of Western society; it is considered an indication to initiate the afflicted person into the spirit dance ceremonial. The spirit dance initiation has been reworked into a collective therapeutic process involving physical, didactic, and psychological methods to induce an altered state of consciousness, leading to the initiate's "rebirth as a true Indian person" (Jilek 1982).

For many North American Indians, who had been indoctrinated throughout their youth in the Indian residential school system, the revival of supposedly "pagan" aboriginal ceremonials created a dilemma. They felt they had to choose between adhering to the heritage of their people or to the Western and Christian values they had been taught to accept as superior, despite their suffering from discrimination and deprivation in Western society.

The Beginning: Gently Engaging the Patient

Irene was a 46-year-old woman of Coast Salish Indian background. She had been treated primarily for arthritis and secondarily for depression by her general practitioner, who referred her to a Euro-Canadian psychiatrist. Irene had been twice widowed and was now married to her third husband, 10 years her junior, who pursued a "native" lifestyle; he was often away hunting and fishing with his friends. Irene had five children from previous marriages and five with her present husband. They lived on a small Coast Salish Indian reservation in the Fraser River Valley of British Columbia, Canada. Irene was struggling to keep house for her large family in an overcrowded and dilapidated home.

Irene was a small woman; she looked older than her 46 years. Leaning heavily on a cane, she walked slowly with obvious pain. Sitting down in the psychiatrist's office, she crossed her hands tensely over the cane handle. Her fingers were grossly deformed by arthritis. Her face had a fearful expression; she hardly lifted her eyes from the floor, avoiding eye contact with the therapist. She did not speak spontaneously; she answered questions hesitatingly, with only a few words, in a low voice, nearly a whisper. In a moment of silence after questions, she began to cry.

The therapist knew that, for most Indian people in the area, contact with a psychiatrist is associated with fears, or even experiences, of being apprehended by police and sent to the mental hospital, and that psychiatric interviews are commonly likened to interrogations by police officers. To make the patient feel more comfortable, it was necessary to avoid appearing as an interrogator and to show a simple human reaction to her emotional pain by giving her time to get hold of herself.

Irene was left to cry for a while to show respect for her feelings and also to give the therapist time to think of a way of putting the patient at ease. When Irene's crying abated, she was asked whether the arthritis caused her much pain. Her attention turned away from the routine psychiatric enquiry to medical, and therefore emotionally less threatening, problems. Irene responded that the physical pain often made her cry. This was accepted as a plausible explanation to avoid any embarrassment for the patient.

For a while, the dialogue was concentrated on her chronic arthritis: how long she had already suffered, what medication she was taking, and whether she had other physical symptoms. She now readily talked about how the arthritis made it difficult for her to do the necessary housework. She said that she often had headaches and had a hard time sleeping at night. The psychiatrist indicated that her general physician would be contacted in order to discuss, and perhaps improve, the treatment regimen. When the psychiatrist touched Irene's crippled fingers and expressed astonishment about how she was able to do her housework with them, the manifestation of empathy elicited a quick smile from the patient.

Now Irene's apprehension was overcome, and she could be induced to talk about her daily life. With some encouragement, she shared her worries about the children. Some of the older teenagers used street drugs and were in trouble with the police, one of her teenage daughters was pregnant, and another had dropped out of school—a sad picture often encountered among the young North American Indian generation in this and other areas. It was rare that the youngsters ever helped Irene in the house, but all expected to be fed and have their laundry done. Irene's husband, rarely at home, had little authority over the youngsters. Sometimes Irene would be afraid of her big sons demanding things she could not provide; their anger would keep her in a state of anxious tension.

These revelations provided enough material for further enquiry and gave the therapist a first picture of Irene's difficult life, illustrating again the common psychosocial stressors facing North American Indian people who live on poverty-stricken reservations. Communicating these problems to a therapist who was listening with interest and empathy allowed the patient to find some comfort in the interview situation.

Already in the second session, which started in a more relaxed atmosphere, Irene related an event that seemed to be of great importance to her. One evening not long before, when driving home, she was stopped by police because of unsteady driving. She had perhaps taken too many painkillers, and when she stumbled out of the car, the officers, assuming she was under the influence of alcohol, arrested her and placed her in the "drunk tank." No explanation or protest helped. Overwhelmed by shame, pain, and sorrow, Irene cried in her cell. When her crying turned into a strange sing-song, the officers thought she was mentally disturbed and expedited her to the mental hospital, where she was diagnosed to have a psychotic depression. Within 2 weeks, and after a few electroshock treatments, she was discharged home, feeling even more upset than before.

Having listened to Irene's recent experience at the police station and the mental hospital, when she first felt stereotyped as a "drunken Indian" and then was taken for a "crazy person" in another humiliating encounter with "white" authority figures, the psychiatrist knew Irene would have to be helped to overcome the resistance she was bound to feel toward a non-Indian therapist. She would have to be encouraged to express her pent-up frustration and resentment and, in spite of her anger, to feel fully accepted as a person by the psychiatrist, before a meaningful therapeutic relationship could be established.

During the weekly sessions that followed, Irene became much more relaxed. The sessions always began with the psychiatrist inquiring whether the prescribed antidepressant and anxiolytic medication had brought some relief. Such inquiries helped Irene to overcome her initial apprehension. Irene was then able to speak about her deep hurt and anger when she was unjustly accused of being drunk and taken into custody. She emphasized that she had never been drunk in her whole life, although she had been under pressure, first by her mother, and then by her husbands, sons, and other relatives, to join drinking parties. Tearfully, Irene related that she had been unable to make the mental hospital staff understand that her singing in the police cell was not a sign of mental disturbance, but a "spirit song," which had forced itself over her lips as an expression of her hurt. The electroshock treatment did not take away the spirit song as she actually had hoped: "That treatment made me forget nice things and left me with what I wanted to forget." She therefore considered the treatment to be a kind of punishment.

The psychiatrist felt it was too early in therapy to take up the topic of the spirit song that Irene had indicated she rather wanted to get rid of. The patient's full confidence would have to be won before an issue touching upon the secrets of Indian spirit power could be discussed. Even in the area of the Coast Salish Indians, only a few non-Indian people are well informed about the winter spirit dances, which were the most important ceremonials of traditional aboriginal culture. In the past, the Christian missionaries had actively discouraged, and the government had officially outlawed, these "pagan rituals" as incompatible with Christianity and "civilization." The psychiatrist knew that if Irene were to accept her spirit-song power, she would, according to native tradition, be expected to participate in the arduous process of being initiated into the revived traditional Salish winter spirit dances. In Irene's case, this would be very difficult, not only because of her crippling arthritis but also because of the Western education and Christian teaching she had absorbed, and with it a general distaste of so-called "primitive Indian ways." In the following sessions, she was, therefore, encouraged to tell her life story.

Exploration of Irene's Background

As a preschool child, Irene lived with her parents on an Indian reservation. At the age of 7, she was sent to an Indian residential school, with her parents' consent. Nobody explained to the little girl why she was taken from her family home to start school in an unknown place far away. The residential school was administered by nuns, and the children had to obey a strict regimen; they were taught in English only and were forbidden to speak their native tongue. Irene felt rejected by her family and wondered what she had done wrong to deserve being sent away. Even these many years later, she had tears in her eyes when she remembered the loneliness and homesickness she experienced during the first years at the residential school. She experienced feelings of guilt and worthlessness that never really left her. Irene's visits home were also filled with bitterness and resentment. The nuns taught her faith in Christ and cleanliness. When she visited her family on the Indian reservation, she began to feel like a stranger among her own people; she was ashamed because of her mother's drinking and the squalor of the homes.

At 16, when she left school, she could hardly speak her native language. She could not help but resent her family, because they put her to work in a cannery to earn a few dollars that they then spent on alcohol. When her brothers tried to make her join their drinking parties, she left home. At the age of 17, Irene married her first husband, with whom she had three children. While in the hospital, giving birth to her second baby, her first child died of neglect at home, because her husband was away drinking. At the age of 30, he died of tuberculosis. Irene obtained a cleaning job at the local government hospital and earned just enough to scrape by with her children, of whom she had another three by her second husband, who also died young.

She married her third husband, hoping he would be a good provider, but he preferred to roam with his friends rather than to help support her and the five children he eventually fathered. In time, he became a chronic alcohol abuser prone to paranoid jealousy. At the time of her referral, she had 10 sons and daughters, ages 8 to 20.

As her arthritis worsened, Irene had to give up her job at the hospital. She struggled with the social welfare system to secure enough support for her younger children, and she lived in constant fear that they would be apprehended and placed in a distant foster home. Throughout the years, Irene had worked hard to care for her large family and to keep up with the "white man's" standard, as she had learned it from the nuns at the residential school. She had refused to have "fun" drinking with the others. She did not feel at home on the Indian reservation, where she had few friends: "I hate the reservation and the way the people live there; they are so backwards, they think it is still old times, they see only their little world, they drink and dream, and are without ambition. I hate it because I have always tried to be different, tried to look forward, and understand the modern world . . ." But the ongoing traumatic experiences had made Irene resentful, not only against her kin and against life on the Indian reservation, but also against the "white man," who had estranged her from her own people, without offering the help she needed. She sought comfort in the Catholic Church but was too shy to make friends among the "white" parishioners.

In the next session, Irene expressed her ambivalence toward her husband. She said she could understand he preferred the old Indian way of hunting and fishing to working for a "white" boss, but she resented his drinking and his failure to assist her at home, which made it impossible to lift the family out of poverty. She now admitted that all the disappointments throughout the years had caused her to be unfriendly with her husband and impatient with her children. She sighed and again expressed feelings of hopelessness and futility.

At this point, the therapist felt that Irene needed to be encouraged both by word and by deed. For a person living in physical pain and extreme poverty—a situation most Western therapists have never experienced—individual psychotherapy in the classical detached style will not give significant relief, because much of the emotional distress is related to the adversities of a daily struggle for survival. Irene had already provided the therapist with some insight into her difficult life; her disappointment with an inadequate husband, who escaped from his responsibility by drinking with his friends; the worsening of her arthritis due to poor housing conditions; and her anxiety about how to feed and clothe her children.

Irene was commended for not giving up her struggle for a better life for her family and herself. Ways of obtaining more help from social services were discussed with the patient. A joint meeting with her social worker was arranged, and a letter explaining her medical and financial needs was sent to the agency. These steps led to more effective material support for Irene and her children; they also increased her confidence in the therapist's genuine desire to help her.

Bringing Irene's Supernatural Beliefs Into the Therapy

During one of the next sessions, Irene was talking of her Salish Indian heritage. She mentioned that she had heard the therapist had been invited to attend traditional ceremonials at the longhouse, and she probingly asked what the therapist thought of the "heathen" winter spirit dances.

The psychiatrist realized that, by raising this question, Irene signaled her readiness to discuss the matter of her spirit song and the whole issue of the cultural conflict in which she found herself.

The psychiatrist related to Irene the observation that several Salish Indian persons who had become spirit dancers were able to stay away from alcohol and drug use as they regained self-confidence and again experienced pride in their North American Indian culture. He also noted that, by expressing their emotions in song and dance, women seemed to find solace, and men seemed to overcome feelings of anger and aggression.

The psychiatrist remained nonjudgmental and did not give a personal opinion on beliefs in supernatural powers, but related an observation regarding positive effects of the traditional native ceremonial.

After a long and thoughtful silence, Irene began to talk of her spirit song, which always came to her in an emotional crisis. She admitted that hearing her spirit song, and having to sing it out, scared her very much. The fear that the "spirit-song power" might overwhelm her and force her into spirit dance initiation increased her isolation on the Indian reservation, as she avoided contacts, especially with spirit dancers. Each time her spirit song came, she would be afraid, and her heart would pound wildly. When hearing the drums from the longhouse, she felt they were calling her to the spirit dances; she would jump in the car and drive away. She never wanted to become a spirit dancer. She had tried so hard to live a Christian life; now, to have to sing the "old heathen Indian song" was like a curse to her and made her feel sinful: "I am afraid that I could suddenly die and be on the wrong side."

In the following sessions, Irene was able to express the ambivalent feelings underlying her indecision regarding what to do about her spirit song. It became clear that Irene felt isolated on the reservation and that she longed to be fully accepted by her fellow Indians. But she resented the pressure exerted on her to follow the call of her spirit song and become a spirit dancer. She was reluctant, not only because of her Christian upbringing but also because of the physical pain the dancing in the longhouse would cause her.

The psychiatrist came to the realization that helping the patient overcome her alienation and cultural identity confusion would be essential in resolving her problems of low self-esteem and alleviating her depression. This would be facilitated if the patient became aware that the therapist recognized that traditional healing procedures could be of value and that, by respecting native elders, the therapist showed a positive regard for North American Indian cultures. The psychiatrist knew that sometimes a traditional Salish Indian healer could free a person from an unwanted spirit song if there was a valid reason, one that was acceptable according to native traditions. The psychiatrist decided to bring this up in a session.

A Therapeutic Strategy:
Recommending a Traditional Intervention

As expected, Irene was astonished when presented with a traditional intervention as a possible way out of her dilemma. She found it hard to believe that a modern psychiatrist—one of the physicians whom she regarded as an authority figure of the "white" establishment—would expect any benefit from the intervention of an indigenous healer. However, after some hesitation, she agreed to have the psychiatrist write a letter to a Salish Indian elder in another reservation, who was well known for his shamanic healing.

In this letter, the psychiatrist explained Irene's suffering and the need for a combined effort by both a modern and a traditional therapist to help her. When a very positive response came from the healer, Irene was moved by the warm words of this elder, his interest in her problems, and his offer of help. He wrote that if she came to his place together with family members, he would perform the traditional ceremony to take the spirit song away from her. Irene still hesitated, fearing a negative reaction from her family. The psychiatrist therefore asked her to bring her husband and some of her older children to a joint session so that he could explain the situation and solicit their cooperation.

At this joint family session, Irene appeared surprised at her husband's understanding attitude and the family's expressed readiness to help her. The psychiatrist observed that Irene's husband, a soft-spoken man, was somewhat intimidated by her but was quite interested in the prospect of having a traditional Salish Indian ceremony performed. A date was set for the family's journey to the healer's reservation.

Irene did not come for another appointment until some time after the ceremony had taken place. She was in a cheerful mood; her general condition appeared improved. Without hesitation, she spoke about the healing ceremony that had lasted for many hours into the night. She did not recall details but said a great burden had been lifted off her mind. She was convinced her spirit song would not return. Moreover, she now had won a new and much more positive view of her family members, especially of her husband, who had stood by her side throughout the ceremony. She now welcomed further joint sessions.

From then on, the therapeutic relationship with the psychiatrist was firmly established. It was possible for Irene to explore and candidly express the feelings of cultural identity confusion that had troubled her since her days at the residential school. She relived and abreacted the sadness and rejection she had felt upon separation from her parents and family, when she was taken to the residential school, and her disappointment and embarrassment on home visits later on. She realized how resentment and ambivalence had negatively influenced her significant relationships. She worked through her conflicting feelings about traditional North American Indian and "white" Christian values, and arrived at a positive synthesis that met her emotional needs. The alleviation of Irene's depressed mood allowed her to undergo, with confidence, corrective surgical treatment of her arthritic deformities. The overall betterment of her emotional and physical condition was a great delight to herself and her family. She successfully encouraged her husband to obtain a job and persuaded him that "drinking is not Indian." Their relationship improved, and, with renewed energy, Irene finally felt secure in providing her family with the decent home of which she had always dreamed.

Some time after psychotherapy had been terminated, the psychiatrist received a letter from Irene, in which she wrote:

> Dear Doctor . . . I realize what I could have gotten into but thanks doctor, when I was at my worst you were always there, that was my strength so I managed to keep things under control. You see you're the only one that knew the help I needed. My family didn't realize this or didn't want to. Maybe it is my own fault for hiding it but gosh it made me sick. I'm not so bad now, I don't have many depressive moments, I have learnt to pin what starts me off and try to avoid them, instead try to be happy. Bill [her husband] is working now, I feel more hope for the future. Hope to hear from you. So long! — Irene.

Analysis and Discussion

Ethnic Transference in Intercultural Psychotherapy

Intercultural psychotherapy, as it was termed by Hsu and Tseng (1972), presents a challenge to the Western-trained psychiatrist. This becomes especially apparent in the psychotherapy of North American Indian patients by professionals who are members of the majority society, as demonstrated in this case. To many North American Indian patients, the encounter with the psychiatrist is initially perceived as yet another confrontation with, and interrogation by, a representative of the "white" establishment, whom they expect to be critical of Indian ways, and who has the power to commit people to a psychiatric hospital unit against their will.

Urban Western people have a notion of what psychotherapy is about and are usually quite willing to respond to the therapist's questions. But to Irene, the psychiatrist was initially a "white" authority figure who reminded her of recent fearful experiences with the police and in the mental hospital. This filled her with apprehension, and she was unable to engage in a dialogue and ended up crying. Although wanting help, many North American Indian patients, who have become sensitive to negative comments on Indian behavior, may hesitate to reveal their personal and emotional problems to a "white" professional and may be more concerned with making a good impression on the interviewer. The therapist, on the other hand, frustrated by the lack of meaningful communication, and perhaps also annoyed over, say, unpunctual attendance, will consider the patient "unmotivated" and will soon subscribe to the frequently stated notion that North American Indians are unsuitable candidates for "insight-directed" psychotherapy.

Dealing With Spiritual Beliefs

Dealing with matters of spiritual and religious beliefs is a challenge to the psychotherapist, especially when the patient comes from a different cultural background. With patients in whose ethnic-cultural group traditional healing is practiced, the therapist should strive to expand his or her horizon, beyond the confines of the naturalistic orientation of medical school training, to an understanding of the symbolic meaning of beliefs in the power of supernatural entities and ritual acts, for these are manifestations of sentiments that cannot be judged by the criteria of positive science. The therapist should also be aware that in most non-Western societies, even in urban areas, traditional therapeutic resources continue to be used, especially for patients with psychiatric disorders for which traditional healing has a proven efficacy (Jilek 1993). The onus is on the psychiatrist, who sees patients from a tradition-directed, non-Western background in psychotherapy, to inform himself or herself on the world view and belief system of the patient's culture, as relevant to health and disease. This information can be gathered from the patients themselves; from older family members; from other key informants, such as elders and healers; and from pertinent ethnographic literature. It is of great advantage if the therapist can obtain the cooperation of indigenous traditional practitioners who are likely to be involved. When a tradition-directed, non-Western patient is geographically isolated from culture-congenial resources and has to be seen in modern psychotherapy— as distinct from symptomatic medical-psychiatric treatment—the patient should be looked upon as the key informant on his or her culture and should be given the opportunity of sharing his or her traditional belief system with an unbiased and interested therapist.

Bridging the Cultural Gap Between Therapist and Patient

The psychiatrist in the case report had obtained, from literature and personal contacts with tribal elders, the information on the history and the understanding of traditional beliefs and customs of the area's indigenous population, which is indispensable for psychotherapy with North American Indian patients. The psychiatrist already had experience with North American Indian patients and, therefore, knew that, in these cases, interviewing strategy and technique had to be modified by initially focusing attention on general health and socioeconomic problems. Because Irene, besides being depressed, suffered from painful arthritis, the psychiatrist neutralized the tense interview situation by interpreting her crying as due to her pain, whereupon the patient readily talked about her physical complaints. As in many other cases involving North American Indian patients, the social and financial plight of Irene and her children significantly contributed to her mental state.

The psychiatrist's unsolicited intervention with the responsible social service agency on the patient's behalf went a long way toward creating a relationship of trust and would have been of therapeutic significance, even if it had not resulted in material benefits. Very often, difficulties in establishing a therapeutic relationship with a North American Indian patient are rooted in differences of cultural value orientation, in the history of the "Indian-white" relationship, and in the patient's own experience of this relationship. Whereas modern Western people usually believe in individual solutions, give priority to individualistic concerns, limit their social obligations to those of the nuclear family, and view having children as neither absolutely necessary nor universally desirable, many North American Indians still believe in group solutions, feel a strong obligation toward their kin, and consider having children an absolute necessity and universally desirable. Whereas modern Western people try to avoid long-term commitments to others outside their immediate family, and consider participation in ceremonial group functions as voluntary and dispensable, many North American Indians feel bound to such commitments and to honor ceremonial functions.

Irene's life story demonstrated her strong feelings of obligation toward her spouses and her many children, in spite of their often reckless and aggressive behavior, which among members of the dominant society would, as a rule, lead to family breakup. Some Western therapists might even counsel such a solution, in view of the hardships Irene had suffered from her family. However, this was not a solution that Irene could have accepted, because of her tradition-bound sense of solidarity with her kin group.

Involving the Family

It is generally helpful, in most psychotherapeutic situations, to have at least one joint informative session with family members or significant others. In psychotherapy with tradition-directed, non-Western patients, it is essential to involve the family in the therapeutic process. Since Irene had been hesitant to have a joint session with her family members, because she felt they lacked understanding of her situation, the psychiatrist was looking for a suitable occasion to draw the husband and some of her older children into the therapeutic process. This opportunity eventually presented itself, because the family's cooperation was requested by the traditional healer. The positive attitude shown by her husband and children during joint sessions surprised Irene and led to marked improvement in the intrafamily situation and in the patient's emotional condition.

Resolving Acculturation Stress

Unlike many North American Indians, a psychiatrist coming from the majority society has no personal experience of acculturation stress. Only if the psychiatrist succeeds in establishing a therapeutic trust relationship will the North American Indian patient reveal experiences and emotions that have to do with what has been called the "core complex" (Jilek-Aall 1978), the cluster of feeling-toned ideas associated with the "Indian-white" relationship, as perceived or experienced by the patient: anger about social discrimination, frustration due to cultural identity confusion, grief about the disappearance of native language and traditions because of previous suppression, resentment generated by relative deprivation, and shame over the obvious examples of moral degradation due to abuse of intoxicants, originally introduced by "whites."

Irene's struggle with this core complex was revealed as soon as she opened up to tell her personal experiences since childhood. She was taken away at an early age from her native environment, and throughout her formative years Western behavioral norms and Christian values were imposed on her, through rigid indoctrination at the residential school. At the same time, her people's customs and traditions were denigrated as "heathen" and "primitive," and the use of her native language was forbidden. "Proper" conduct and cleanliness were inculcated into the child, but love and acceptance were not shown by her strict caregivers. Irene developed a strong resentment against "white" majority society, which was reinforced every time she had to report to, or deal with, agents of this society, such as social workers, schoolteachers, police officers, and other authority figures. However, Irene also tried to aspire to the standards of "white" society, as the nuns had impressed them upon her, especially in terms of cleanliness and proper behavior. She did not feel comfortable on the Indian reservation, where she saw poverty, squalor, and alcohol-induced deviant and aggressive behavior that threatened to degrade her own children. Irene had identified this kind of lifestyle with "Indian ways," just as her prejudiced educators had done, when, in fact, it reflected decades of social deterioration due to the systematic destruction of aboriginal culture under past governmental and ecclesiastic policies.

Irene eventually became aware of the value of traditional Salish Indian culture, when the therapist encouraged her to learn from tribal elders and to undergo a traditional healing ceremony, with the assistance of her family.

Irene was able to find a resolution to the frustrating culture conflict caused by her core complex, when a firmly established psychotherapeutic relationship allowed her to use traditional resources without abandoning her Christian beliefs.

References

Benedict RF: The concept of the guardian spirit in North America. Memoirs of the American Anthropological Association, No 29, 1923

Hsu J, Tseng WS: Intercultural psychotherapy. Arch Gen Psychiatry 27:700–705, 1972

Jilek WG: Salish Indian Mental Health and Culture Change. Toronto, Holt, Rinehart & Winston, 1974

Jilek WG: Native renaissance: the survival and revival of indigenous therapeutic ceremonials among North American Indians. Transcultural Psychiatric Research Review 15:117–147, 1978

Jilek WG: Indian Healing: Shamanic Ceremonialism in the Pacific Northwest Today. Surrey, BC, Hancock House Publishers, 1982

Jilek WG: Traditional medicine relevant to psychiatry, in Treatment of Mental Disorders: A Review of Effectiveness. Edited by Sartorius N, de Girolamo G, Andrews G, et al. Washington, DC, American Psychiatric Press, 1993, pp 341–383 (published on behalf of the World Health Organization)

Jilek-Aall L: Alcohol and the Indian-White relationship: a study of the function of Alcoholics Anonymous among Coast Salish Indians. Confinia Psychiatrica 21: 195–233, 1978

CHAPTER 5

The Woman Who Alienated Her Family After Losing Her Son

Alan A. Buffenstein, M.D.

Case Report

This case involves the therapy of a middle-aged woman who was having difficulty accepting the tragic death of her son. There was a cultural gap between therapist and patient, and their relationship was key to a successful outcome. As the case is presented in this chapter, observations on the case by the treating psychiatrist are represented by the paragraphs in italics.

Mariko Smith: The Patient

Mrs. Mariko Smith, a 56-year-old, married Japanese American female, sought treatment with a psychiatrist following a panic attack in a store. For several weeks, she had been increasingly tense, with difficulty concentrating and an inability to sleep at night. Mrs. Smith was a *nisei* (i.e., second-generation Japanese American) who had never seen a psychiatrist before. She previously had been high-functioning and employed, drove her own car, and was a homemaker. Searching through the local telephone book, she carefully chose a therapist who was not Japanese. She told the psychiatrist that her only son had been killed, "murdered," by a careless drunk driver 2 months previously. She persistently ruminated over this event, even vividly imagining various scenarios about how the death actually occurred.

The Therapist

The psychiatrist, a 35-year-old Jewish man, had been trained in the United States but raised in other countries. He was new to Hawaii, a place notable for its mixture of ethnicities and cultures. He had just started his private practice, and his interview room had not yet been properly set up. As a result, he was forced to interview Mariko in a large room with his receptionist nearby, behind a partition. He was not pleased about this office arrangement, with its awkwardness. Mariko Smith was extremely polite, well groomed, intelligent, and quite attractive for her age. She was clearly suffering, although she was not attempting to elicit sympathy. Thus, he was particularly concerned, even embarrassed, about the informality of his office setting. But Mrs. Smith, it seemed, was not bothered by the situation. She talked comfortably and was entirely responsive to the therapist's questions as he took her history.

Although her appearance and ethnic background were obviously different, she reminded the therapist of his own mother, who had passed away 3 years previously. It was as if Mrs. Smith were sensitive to *his* needs, making him feel comfortable, despite her own problems. The therapist found her very appealing and found himself quite eager to help her. A contract was established, and the therapist agreed to treat Mrs. Smith. She declined the offer for anti-anxiety medication. She would come for weekly 50-minute sessions, and, in the meantime, she would call if she needed to.

The therapist began to formulate a working hypothesis. This case involved more than simple bereavement. Mrs. Smith appeared on the surface to be very proper, as if she did not want to cause the therapist any distress. Underneath, however, she was overwhelmed and was increasingly isolating herself with her grief. She was alienating herself from her family. Why did she not join her husband and children in their grief so that they could all take comfort in one another and provide solace to each other? The therapist needed to understand more about the patient's relationship with her dead son and with each other member of the family. Perhaps cultural factors were involved, interfering with the communication between husband and wife. Would such factors also influence the therapist-patient relationship?

Reaction to Her Son's Death

The first few sessions elaborated and clarified the reaction of Mrs. Smith to the tragic loss of her son. She had initially responded to the news about her son's death with disbelief. Then, several days after hearing the news, she had experienced a terrible pain in her head, like an explosion. After that, she tended to lose her sense of time and interest in her usual activities and was unable to discern meaning in her life. After the incident, the patient would retire to her room with little communication with her family, leaving them to their own devices, not cooking or spending any time with them. She and her husband found themselves like strangers, walking by each other, saying little. She described herself as numb, devoid of feelings for her husband.

Mrs. Smith could not stop thinking about her son. She kept reliving his funeral, focusing on small details that were seemingly insignificant but greatly bothersome to her. Certain details had not been attended to properly, or at least not to her satisfaction. Her husband and two daughters had dismissed her concerns as inconsequential. This infuriated her; it was as if they were devaluing her son.

The only activity she permitted herself revolved around continuing her son's work as a martial arts instructor. She felt dutybound to attend the group's tournaments, as if she were fulfilling her son's obligation. Her family wanted her to stop attending these events and to join them in other activities. To her, this demonstrated their lack of understanding. Yet she wanted them to go on about their own business; she certainly did not want them to join her at the tournaments.

She verbalized fears of going crazy. She had reached the end of her rope and was particularly worried about her potential for losing emotional control in public. If she were to show her feelings, this would result in her being locked up in a mental hospital, and her life would end at that point. She became hypervigilant, lest she give herself away.

She had frequent, powerful fantasies of getting revenge for the traffic accident of her son. These fantasies were being stimulated by an impending court case associated with her son's death. Mrs. Smith was terrified, and quite embarrassed, that she might become enraged in court at the sight of the perpetrator and experience an overwhelming desire to kill the man who had "murdered" her son. She was thinking about this when she had the panic attack in the store.

Mariko Smith's Life History

As therapy progressed, the patient's personal history gradually became clear. Mariko Fujikami had married a Caucasian man, Charles Smith, 35 years ago.

They had three children, the oldest being her 32-year-old son, now deceased. He had not married and had had no serious relationship, although he had been socially active with friends. The Smiths had two daughters, ages 24 and 21. The older daughter was married and lived nearby. The younger daughter was finishing college and still lived at home. There were no grandchildren.

Mrs. Smith described herself as coming from a traditional Japanese background; her parents had both immigrated to Hawaii from Japan, and Japanese was still spoken in their home. They also observed Japanese festivals and tended to eat Japanese food. Mrs. Smith was one of two daughters and several sons. Her father was a schoolteacher and her mother was a homemaker. She was close to her parents, and while growing up, she seemed to enjoy a special relationship with her father. As a young adult, she rebelled against her conservative Japanese family, and at the age of 22 she married a Caucasian military man. Her parents, although comfortable within their Western setting, were strongly against the interracial marriage, and by disobeying them, she had alienated her family. They had shown coolness toward her *haole* (white) husband and practically ignored their racially mixed grandson for many years.

When the granddaughters came along, the Fujikami's softened somewhat, but the relationship between Mrs. Smith and her mother remained distant and strained. In her last years, the mother suffered from dementia and eventually had to live in a nursing home. The patient, as a filial daughter, had fulfilled her obligations by frequently visiting her mother, but her mother remained cool to her until the end. Her mother died a year before the present treatment, and Mrs. Smith reported that she had not been too saddened by this and had accepted the death as natural and inevitable.

Her husband's family, living in another state, had also been against their marriage and had never really taken an interest in the couple's children. Over the years, Mrs. Smith experienced disappointment with her husband, and they came to live fairly separate lives. He spent time with his golfing friends, but she preferred to be with her children, especially her deceased son, to whom she was very attached.

Process of Therapy

At the initiation of therapy, Mrs. Smith was very tense, like a coiled-up spring ready to release. She had the notion that she was numb and dissociated from her own feelings and behaviors and that there was so much anger under the surface that if she could experience her feelings, then the forces holding them in would break loose, resulting in chaos. On several occasions, she phoned between sessions, experiencing panic-like anxiety. The calls were always brief, and Mrs. Smith was always very appreciative. Unlike some patients, she was never demanding or imposing.

The therapist found himself being very gentle with Mrs. Smith, as if he were reflecting back her tendency to be polite and solicitous. The therapist was sensitive to the possibility of a transference reaction in which the patient might idealize him and denigrate her husband, unconsciously seeking to replace her lost son or her husband with the therapist. The patient maintained her boundaries, however, always being quite proper, and the therapist chose not to make any such interpretation.

He considered having Mr. Smith join the therapy. Her husband must be grieving also, and it would certainly help if they could grieve together, providing mutual support. The therapist did not even bring up this idea, however, and he reflected on why he did not. He enjoyed these sessions with Mrs. Smith, and he did not want to interrupt the process. At first he felt guilty about this. How could he feel such a strong bond with this patient, who was so culturally different from himself? He had no erotic feelings toward Mrs. Smith, and he sensed none coming from her. Gradually he realized that she did not see him as a replacement for her husband, but more as the son she had lost. And she evoked feelings in him of his own mother. He did not interpret any of this for the patient, particularly since she seemed to be getting better.

Although the therapist did not notice it at first, Mrs. Smith developed a relationship with his receptionist, a first-generation Filipino woman. Mrs. Smith would even call the receptionist to get advice and yet would never bring this up with the therapist. Mrs. Smith gradually seemed to enjoy her sessions, simultaneously with the extra contact with the receptionist. It was as if she had developed a surrogate family to which she could retreat—one in which there were no duties or obligations, and in which she was uncritically accepted, and even encouraged to share her fears and worries. The therapist initially worried about the contact with the receptionist, but again, since Mrs. Smith was getting better, he did not say anything.

At the suggestion of the therapist, Mrs. Smith got involved in new activities and stopped going to the martial arts tournaments. She would discuss her new activities with the therapist. He took great interest in all of this, and his interest encouraged Mrs. Smith to continue her new involvements.

As time progressed, an impending court case involving prosecution of the drunk driver became a focus in therapy. Mrs. Smith wanted to attend the trial, but she feared she would fall apart. The trial coincided with the anniversary of her son's death. Her nightmares returned, and, once again, she became preoccupied with trivial details associated with her son's death and his funeral. She expressed great disappointment with her husband for his behavior through all this.

The therapist used this opportunity to shift the focus of therapy toward Mrs. Smith's relationship with her husband. He pointed out how bold and strong she must have been to marry him against her parents' wishes, especially because she had always been, and remained, an exceptionally dutiful daughter. The therapist told Mrs. Smith that he wished he could be as good a son as she had been a daughter. This seemed to have a powerful effect on Mrs. Smith. She became tearful and told the therapist that she was certain no son could be better than him. At this point, the therapist sensed that Mrs. Smith was beginning to come to terms with the loss of her own son. Indeed, she was able to attend the trial and maintain her composure.

The therapist also suggested that because of the exceptional boldness and courage that it took to marry her *haole* husband, she must have had great expectations for him, which he could not possibly meet. This led to discussions that proved quite fruitful over the next few sessions. It seems that Mrs. Smith was originally attracted to her husband because he was so different from her parents. She envisioned a more liberated lifestyle with him. Over time, however, she became very disappointed in him. They could never communicate well. He seemed incapable of even basic Japanese-style courtesies. She could never admit her disappointment to her parents. She could tolerate the disappointments in her own life, however, because of her son. She devoted her life to him, and this gave her sustenance. After these issues were clarified in therapy, Mrs. Smith seemed much more at peace with herself. She developed increasing interest in her daughters and resumed socializing with friends. With mutual agreement, the therapy was ended with reasonable satisfaction.

Throughout the nearly 1-year course of therapy, the patient was always compliant, nicely groomed, punctual for her appointments, and prompt in paying her bill. She established a positive relationship of trust with the therapist and developed a strong dependency on the therapy. Mrs. Smith stated that the sessions provided her with much relief and, indeed, were her lifeline. She perceived the therapist as always being there for her in her hour of need.

As a whole, the therapist afforded the patient strengthening by providing empathy and accepting interpersonal dependency. Letting her speak freely, being noncritical, and being available to her to help her express her fears and anger without the concern of losing face provided her a forum within which the grieving process became freed up. With improvement, she began to experience a return of her emotions in a manageable manner. The marriage remained cool, but the patient was less angry and more accepting of her husband the way he was.

Analysis and Discussion

Stereotypes About Asian Patients and Intercultural Therapy

It is a commonly held stereotype that, because of stigma, Asian patients are reluctant to seek psychotherapy, and that even if they did they would have difficulty using it to examine their psychological life. However, the case presented here suggests otherwise. Despite her Asian background, Mariko Smith was able to make good use of psychotherapy to her great benefit.

It is also a commonly held notion that many obstacles exist when the therapist and patient have different racial and/or cultural backgrounds. Yet, in this case, the difference was probably advantageous. Mariko Fujikami married Charles Smith partly because she was rebelling against the strict culture of her parents. She needed a non-Japanese therapist to validate that it was okay to have a serious relationship with a man from another culture, despite her parents' disapproval. Because of her cultural upbringing, as well as her character structure, she maintained formality and correct boundaries with the therapist, but their relationship was extremely meaningful, even intimate, from her perspective, since she had shared thoughts and feelings that she had not even shared with her husband (Lebra 1984). Thus, in this case, it may have been advantageous that the patient and therapist had different ethnic backgrounds. It required that the therapist be sensitive to cultural differences and flexible enough to make adjustments for the patient.

Interview Setting: The Matter of Privacy

The therapist by training and personal cultural background placed importance in having privacy and confidentiality in psychotherapy, so he was naturally concerned about the relatively open space where he conducted therapy with Mariko Smith—with his receptionist sitting nearby. In retrospect, this undesirable setting may actually have been helpful. The value of privacy differs across cultures. Mrs. Smith had been raised in a Japanese home where privacy was not emphasized, and she did not expect privacy in the same way the therapist did. Furthermore, having a third person, particularly a woman, nearby may have provided a buffering effect for Mrs. Smith, mitigating the concern that she was revealing personal matters to a stranger and being overly close with a man outside her family.

Connection to the Receptionist

The therapist expected the patient to have minimal interaction with the receptionist. This was consistent both with his psychoanalytic training and with the society in which he grew up, which stressed the importance of individualism. In contrast, the (Asian) culture of the Fujikami's emphasizes more interdependence among family and close associates (Doi 1973). Thus, Mrs. Smith considered it culturally quite natural and appropriate for her, as a female, to relate to the female receptionist, who was quite outgoing and inviting. In her mind, she may have seen the receptionist not merely as a receptionist for the office, but as a family-type extension of the therapist. While disconcerted by their relationship, the therapist realized that, in this particular case, it was actually helpful to the therapy.

Mitigating the Pain of Loss

People from different ethnic backgrounds may vary in their perceptions of the meaning of death and reactions to it. Culture can influence the grief process through culturally prescribed mourning patterns and preferential coping styles (Kalish and Reynolds 1981; Rosenblatt 1993). In Mariko Smith's case, her grief was more intense as a result of the tragic, senseless manner in which the loss occurred, but her difficulty in grieving also had strong cultural influences. In Japanese culture, the mother-son relationship is very close, and the oldest son has a special position of privilege, both because he is culturally designated to become the next head of the family and because the father leaves the upbringing of the children to the mother. A close mother-son relationship is culturally accepted under the notion of filial piety. In Mrs. Smith's case, her feelings for her favored son seem to have been overdetermined, secondary to her own parents' coolness toward her mixed-race son, and her dissatisfaction with her husband. In this case, the therapist served as a replacement for the son, filling an emotional vacuum.

An Acceptable Forum for Dealing With Negative Emotions

Mariko Smith was a *nisei,* or second-generation Japanese American, a generation at high risk for acculturation stress because of the value change between cultures—from traditional Japanese to Western. In Japanese culture, social qualities of forbearance and restraint (*enryo*) are valued to the point where public display of anger is discouraged, particularly for a female. Feelings of anger are understood and accepted, but the public expression of such feelings is not. In the case of Mrs. Smith, the lack of understanding on the part of her husband and the lack of support on the part of her parents contributed to both her anger and her overwhelming fear of its expression. The therapy provided the opportunity to examine and deal with this cultural limitation on the expression of negative emotion, which needed to be identified before Mrs. Smith could successfully grieve and allow herself to move on.

Role of the Therapist

In her time of need, Mariko Smith remained alienated from her family. She could not allow her family of origin to provide emotional support, even if they were capable of it, because she did not expect their support to be unqualified. She was too angry with her husband to share her grief with him. And she was too guilty about favoring her son to burden her daughters. Therefore, it became crucial that the therapist provided a nonjudgmental, supportive relationship, which he carefully maintained in a professional manner so that the patient would not be threatened by feeling too close to him. The appropriate closeness between therapist and patient is determined by the type of therapy (within professional standards) and also must match acceptable norms as defined by the patient's culture. This issue of appropriate level of closeness is particularly critical in intercultural therapy, and it is one area that is vulnerable to being overlooked, with adverse effects on the therapy.

Transcultural Empathy

The context in which a Jewish therapist is treating a Japanese American patient may on the surface suggest a considerable cultural gap, yet a transethnic common value system involving family ties and the mother-son relationship may be shared by both therapist and patient (Herz and Rosen 1982). The transference reaction of Mariko Smith made her respond to the therapist as if he were a good son. The therapist found that she evoked in him memories of his own mother. Fantasizing what his mother's reaction to his own death in similar circumstances would have been like allowed him to more readily empathize with his patient's feelings. Although culturally influenced, human emotions are universal, and empathy may be established across a cultural gap.

References

Doi T: The Anatomy of Dependence: The Key Analysis of Japanese Behavior. Tokyo, Kodansha International, 1973

Herz FM, Rosen EJ: Jewish families, in Ethnicity and Family Therapy. Edited by McGoldrick M, Pearce JK, Giordano J. New York, Guilford, 1982, pp 364–392

Kalish RA, Reynolds DK: Death and Ethnicity: A Psychocultural Study. Farmingdale, NY, Baywood Publishing Company, 1981, pp 120–154

Lebra TS: Japanese Women: Constraint and Fulfillment. Honolulu, University of Hawaii Press, 1984, pp 294–323

Rosenblatt PC: Cross cultural variations in grief: the experience, expression, and understanding of grief, in Ethnic Variations in Dying, Death and Grief. Edited by Irish DP, Lundquist KF, Nelsen VJ. Washington, DC, Taylor & Francis, 1993, pp 13–19

CHAPTER 6

One Patient, Three Therapists

Barry S. Carlton, M.D.

Case Report

This rather unusual case, but one that occurs in clinical practice, involves the therapy of one patient with three therapists, each of whom had different cultural backgrounds and different value systems. It provides a unique opportunity to examine the ways in which culture can influence the psychotherapy process. This case also illustrates three important culturally patterned types of illness behavior: dependency, somatization, and noncompliance.

Mr. Yee: The Patient

A 45-year-old, first-generation Chinese American male, Mr. Yee, presented to a hospital emergency department with his wife. At the time he was tearful and experiencing severe anxiety. He described the feeling of having lost his "face." He did not wish to live anymore. He wanted to "cut off my face and bury it . . . [and] cut myself in the stomach." He had multiple somatic complaints, including headache, pain in the stomach, and weakness of arms and legs. He described a depressed, anxious mood; an inability to sleep; poor appetite with weight loss over the past several weeks; and poor concentration. His history revealed that he had developed severe emotional turmoil several weeks before his emergent presentation. The precipitating event occurred while he was at work. He said his boss yelled at and threatened him in front of his fellow workers. He was afraid he would be fired after an inadequate performance appraisal.

Additional history taken in the emergency room revealed that Mr. Yee, with his wife and daughter, had migrated to the United States from mainland China approximately 10 years before. Initially, he worked in a Chinese restaurant for several years. After he learned to speak some English, he obtained work as a maintenance man for a major hotel chain. He had enjoyed his work and steady income until the event with his boss occurred. There was a previous episode of depression, for which he had been treated with an unknown medication.

He was admitted to the hospital and assigned to a Caucasian psychiatrist, Dr. Jones.

The First Therapist: Dr. Jones

Treatment in the hospital focused on Mr. Yee's overwhelming response to his perceived job difficulty, techniques to remedy the situation, and plans to return to work. Mr. Yee complained that his boss had not been appreciative of his skills and performance and had demoted him. He reported that he had been yelled at and criticized in front of his colleagues. Mr. Yee told Dr. Jones that he had endured considerable hardship when he emigrated from China to the United States. He described how he had acquired special occupational skills and a certificate of training. He took great pride in his work and in his ability to support his family. Dr. Jones took this as evidence of considerable strength of character, suggesting a good prognosis if Mr. Yee could return to work soon.

To assess the reality of the situation, Dr. Jones spoke with the employer. The story he obtained was much different from the one Mr. Yee reported. In fact, there had been no disciplinary action. Instead, the patient's job had been changed to meet the exigencies of the work site. An attempt to help clarify this reality with Mr. Yee was surprisingly (to Dr. Jones) unsuccessful.

Mr. Yee's panic and anxiety were treated with medication. Strategies to help the patient right the felt wrong at work were suggested. All of these, however, involved what the patient was required to do. The emphasis was on improving the patient's instrumental skills and a restoration of his independence and autonomy. Dr. Jones interviewed Mrs. Yee, and she expressed great concern about Mr. Yee's need to return to work and financially support the family. When a discharge date was planned, however, Mr. Yee dramatically collapsed, having what he called a "seizure." The patient stated that the newly prescribed medication was "too strong" for him and that this caused him to faint. Dr. Jones recognized Mr. Yee's desire to be taken care of by the hospital and by Dr. Jones, but this desire was viewed in the context of a pathological regression during acute illness, something to be directly challenged.

Several days later, with a great deal of encouragement, the depression, anxiety, and suicidal ideation ameliorated to the point where Mr. Yee was able to be discharged and return home.

Mr. Yee agreed to follow up with Dr. Jones for outpatient psychotherapy, which emphasized coping strategies for his emotional difficulty. He was reluctant to return to work, however, and there was no resolution of the conflict with his employer. The therapy then focused primarily on helping Mr. Yee return to work. The patient felt that Dr. Jones did not understand his need for having more rest for recuperation. Ultimately, he and his wife requested a change in therapist, stating a language barrier as a problem, despite Mr. Yee's good skills in English.

The Second Therapist: Dr. Chang

The patient and his wife were referred to another psychiatrist, Dr. Chang, whose ethnic origin was Chinese and who spoke Chinese to some extent. Dr. Chang not only practiced psychiatry but also saw general medical patients, which pleased Mr. Yee a great deal, since he expected help for his multiple somatic complaints. The patient knew Dr. Chang, having seen him 2 years earlier for depression. Psychotherapy was carried out in a mixture of Chinese and English. Mr. and Mrs. Yee were pleased that Dr. Chang was able to speak some Chinese, helping them to communicate and complain about problems in their native language. Yet, they ultimately became displeased, because the therapist did not talk very much, did not offer explanations, and "did nothing but listen to complaints."

Dr. Chang felt Mr. Yee was excessively concerned about his body's condition and too easily complained of side effects from his medication. As a result, different medication regimens were tried. The frequent switches in medication were taken by Mr. Yee as a sign that Dr. Chang did not understand his problems well. Mr. Yee remained anxious and depressed and frequently called Dr. Chang by phone, paged him after working hours, and dropped into his office without an appointment. This situation lasted for several months. Mr. Yee disturbed Dr. Chang's clinical practice by appearing without an appointment and remaining for excessively long periods of time. Dr. Chang became increasingly intolerant of his patient's "sticky" attachment and overdependence on him. He finally gave up and referred Mr. Yee to Dr. Tam.

The Third Therapist: Dr. Tam

Dr. Tam was also of Chinese ethnicity. He was described to Mr. Yee as an experienced and well-regarded psychiatrist in the community, one who spoke Mandarin well. Dr. Chang also told Mr. Yee that Dr. Tam was the last resort for him, if he wanted to get well. The psychotherapy was carried out entirely in Mandarin, the language with which the patient felt most comfortable. Mrs. Yee was invited to join the sessions. It was apparent that Mr. Yee relied on his wife greatly and that she could play a significant role in his treatment.

From the start, Dr. Tam told Mr. Yee that he required medication "to improve his brain," because his brain suffered from too great a burden at this time. Knowing that the patient had previously complained about medication and had not taken it as prescribed, Dr. Tam placed great emphasis on how to take the medication and how to deal with the anticipated side effects during careful explanations to both Mr. and Mrs. Yee. A Chinese textbook of psychiatry (written by Dr. Tam) was used to help them understand, and their compliance with the medication regimen was required as a condition of treatment. A sample of the prescribed medication (as a gift from Dr. Tam) was given to start the medication. Although Mr. Yee still vigorously complained of side effects as he had previously, he did follow the order to take the medication. Mr. Yee ultimately responded positively to the antidepressant medication, which was the same one prescribed by Drs. Jones and Chang but that Mr. Yee had not actually taken.

The patient continuously demonstrated excessive dependency. He would call Dr. Tam by phone several times in between his weekly sessions, mainly to present his somatic complaints and to ask for reassurance. His wife also complained that the patient was constantly making somatic complaints to her and to their teenage daughter. The family was becoming intolerant of his illness behavior.

To minimize the disturbance to his daily schedule, and to establish therapeutic boundaries, Dr. Tam made an agreement with Mr. Yee that he could phone and leave a brief message, but the call would not be returned unless Dr. Tam felt it was really a matter of urgency. In subsequent sessions, Mr. Yee would almost ritually start the conversation with a litany of his multiple somatic discomforts. He was then allowed to make his somatic complaints and to vent his suffering for not more than 5 minutes. He was told that the session needed to focus on more important issues. By utilizing Mr. Yee's wife as a co-therapist, Dr. Tam was always able to shift the subject to a discussion of how to help him recover from his illness—for the sake of his wife and daughter.

It was revealed that Mr. Yee had lost his father when he was young, and his sister, who was only 3 years older, had raised him almost completely. His mother had been busy working to support the family and taking care of other children. He said that it was his habit to make complaints to his sister to get her attention. He stated that he hoped Dr. Tam would care for him as his "father." He expressed a wish to obtain as much help and guidance from the therapist as possible. He made multiple excuses to prolong each session. Typically, when the session ended, he tried to bring up a new subject for discussion, standing at the door, not wanting to leave. Dr. Tam explained to Mr. Yee that his needs were understandable, but his excessive dependence on his family members and on his therapist would turn them away from him. He was warned, in a joking way, that he might lose his therapist if he did not learn how to maintain "dependence" in a proper way.

Dr. Tam used his established role as an authority figure, offering support as well as guidance. The patient was advised—through direct interpretation of his behavior, even by teasing or benevolent threatening—to diminish his excessive dependency. He was advised not to nag and complain to his family. He was to save such complaints for the first 5 minutes of each session. Because of his great need to be taken care of by Dr. Tam and to please him, Mr. Yee now, paradoxically, had to become more independent.

At the same time, some dependence was allowed, and Dr. Tam provided "expert" advice. Mr. Yee was told to take "nutritious food" and "tonic herbs" to regain his body "force," and he was encouraged to exercise to regain his body "strength." Mr. Yee constantly complained that he had not regained his previous healthy condition for work. He continuously worried that he might in the future be dismissed at any time by his boss for not working satisfactorily. He was fearful that he could not support his family. By using a Chinese proverb—namely, "If you have a green mountain, you would not worry about food for your life"—Mr. Yee was encouraged to work on the recovery of his health rather than worry about losing his job.

Mr. and Mrs. Yee were quite satisfied with Dr. Tam. They felt listened to and understood and were pleased that Dr. Tam provided advice on how to deal with Mr. Yee's personal life and work. Mr. Yee gradually improved and then decided to return to work.

After a year of treatment, Dr. Tam started to decrease the frequency of sessions for practical reasons, as well as therapeutic intent. Mr. Yee, perhaps feeling that the "weaning" was too soon for him and without discussing it with Dr. Tam, visited other physicians—a neurologist for his headaches, his internist (Dr. Chang) for stomach pains, and the hospital emergency room for dizziness. This attention-seeking behavior was understandable to Dr. Tam, who tried to tolerate it. But Dr. Tam was greatly annoyed when the patient discontinued his medication.

Mr. Yee took a vacation from work and visited his hometown in China. He met his older sister, who had taken care of him when he was young. She commented that "Western medicine" was "too strong" for the brain. He needed traditional Chinese herbal medicine. Mr. Yee followed her suggestion and stopped the medication prescribed by Dr. Tam. One month after his return, his depression recurred. Mr. Yee was then convinced that his brain still needed this "Western medicine."

At this point, however, Dr. Tam was annoyed that the patient, in spite of their previous agreement, had not taken his medication and jeopardized his course of recovery. At the same time, Dr. Tam was planning to be out of town for several months. He took this opportunity to refer Mr. Yee back to Dr. Chang.

Returning to the Second Therapist: Dr. Chang

Mr. Yee was now convinced that he needed to take his medication, which had helped him. Dr. Chang told Mr. Yee that he would see him only briefly, primarily for medication, and would not allow him to disturb his regular clinic schedule. This included not paging him after working hours. Mr. Yee accepted these conditions and faithfully took the medication as prescribed. Mr. Yee seemed content with what he got from Dr. Chang at this point and continued to see him, although occasionally he would have somatic complaints and ask for a physical examination from Dr. Chang as his "internist."

Epilogue

As a result of his illness, Mr. and Mrs. Yee considered whether it would be a better for him to leave his work and search for another job. He constantly felt pressure from the supervisor who had yelled at him. He remained fearful that he would be dismissed at any time.

There was an opportunity for a new Chinese market in the community. Mr. and Mrs. Yee decided that this was a chance to develop a new career where they would be their own bosses. They both quit their jobs, and together they opened a small food store. Their teenage daughter, as well as Mr. Yee's mother-in-law, joined them to look after the store whenever they were available. Surrounded by his family, and having a store of his own, Mr. Yee was happy. He and his wife took comfort in the security of now being able to rely on their own "green mountain," and not needing to fear being fired by others. Mr. Yee still kept asking Dr. Chang when he could discontinue his Western medicine, but he had regained his confidence and ability to function.

Analysis and Discussion

Ethnic Matching of Therapist and Patient

Although the proper matching of a therapist and patient of the same ethnic-cultural background has been advocated, particularly by some minority-focused cultural psychiatrists, this case illustrates that ethnic-cultural matching is not a simple matter. Factors associated with the influence of ethnicity on the patient-therapist fit include stage of treatment, nature of the problems to be dealt with, level of ethnic-cultural issues involved in the case, and the therapist's other clinical attributes beyond the matter of language and ethnic or cultural background.

The case of Mr. Yee illustrates three different approaches, each of which had cultural implications influencing the therapeutic outcome. All three therapists identified the same problems to be treated, and they understood the patient's medication requirements identically. Each therapist, however, approached the patient from a somewhat different point of view. A cultural analysis helps explain the different therapeutic values and the different outcomes encountered.

Dr. Jones

The primary task for Dr. Jones was to help Mr. Yee recover from his acute symptoms, and, in fact, he successfully resolved the immediate crisis. There was a reduction in depression and anxiety, and the suicidal ideation completely disappeared. Mr. Yee was able to return home and agreed to follow up as an outpatient. His hospital stay had been short, because of pressures from his tightly managed insurance program, his wife's desire for a rapid recovery and return to work, and Dr. Jones's therapeutic orientation, which placed particular value on autonomy and personal responsibility.

Outpatient therapy was not successful, however. Antidepressant medication, started in the hospital, was continued, but Mr. Yee feared the medication and rarely took it. Mrs. Yee participated in the outpatient sessions because Mr. Yee insisted that his wife was able to communicate better in English and could speak for him. Dr. Jones attempted to reassure Mr. Yee that his English was idiomatic and excellent, but he was happy to have Mrs. Yee present. He appreciated her common sense and motivation for her husband to recover. In therapy sessions, Mrs. Yee consistently expressed to Dr. Jones her concern about lost income and her strong desire for her husband to return to work, but she carefully avoided directly confronting her husband. Dr. Jones failed to appreciate the meaning of Mr. Yee's wish to have his wife talk for him—that is, the wish for someone else to accept his need to be taken care of and manage his recovery for him.

Dr. Jones was guided by his professional and cultural values that a person needs to actively cope with his or her problems and regain his or her level of function as soon as possible. He perceived the role of the therapist as a collaboration with the patient in attaining this goal. Issues are discussed and recommendations are made, but the expectation is that the patient will choose the course of action. Dependency needs, such as Mr. Yee's, may be present but are thought to be balanced by a desire to be autonomous and independent. Psychological independence or autonomy is the highest stage of development according to Western values and theories of psychology.

Mr. Yee's (unconscious) wish to become dependent upon the hospital and therapist was recognized by Dr. Jones but not reinforced. Therapeutic regression was to be avoided. Dr. Jones presented "expert" opinion, but the patient was responsible for choosing his direction and maintaining responsibility both for his treatment and, ultimately, for his recovery and future. This focus on autonomy was interpreted by this Chinese patient, however, as meaning that Dr. Jones was not (culturally) understanding his needs. Dr. Jones expected and invited disagreement with his opinions, but Mr. Yee was paralyzed by not being able to disagree with the therapist (which would be rude in Chinese culture because of Dr. Jones's status as an American physician), and he could resort only to somatic complaints and, when in extreme need, a "seizure."

Dr. Chang

Even though Dr. Chang had an ethnic background similar to the patient's, his primary language was English, and his ability to communicate through Mr. Yee's mother tongue was limited. Nevertheless, Mr. Yee immediately felt much more comfortable than he had with Dr. Jones. Dr. Chang was much more tolerant of Mr. Yee's dependency and much less assertive in encouraging him to go back to work. After a while, however, Dr. Chang's rather passive and nonauthoritarian role was not satisfactory to the patient, who desired to be benevolently guided by authority, and it was even less satisfactory to Mrs. Yee.

The passive stance carries with it an expectation that the patient will present not just problems but psychological material or "associations" as well. The therapist then understands the meaning of the patient's statement and offers an interpretation. The responsibility for the conduct of the therapy is placed upon the patient. The therapist provides the "holding" or safe environment, in which the patient can express his or her difficulties. This again became a problem for this patient. He was still unable to take responsibility for his own treatment and culturally required the therapist to allow Mr. Yee to become dependent upon him. Although Dr. Chang could tolerate a great deal of dependent behavior, the critical issues were not being resolved, and thus Mr. Yee's demands for attention to his symptoms escalated, until Dr. Chang's tolerance level was passed.

Dr. Chang's style was well suited to the patient's needs when he returned after treatment with Dr. Tam, however. The patient was back at work and had only mild residual symptoms. His demands were minimal, and periodic short visits to Dr. Chang provided the sense of security that sustained him as he made important life decisions. Dr. Chang was comfortable with this degree of dependence.

Dr. Tam

Dr. Tam had the advantage of communicating with Mr. Yee in his primary language. It certainly made the communication much more meaningful and effective from a cultural perspective. Understanding the nuances of language was critical to the psychotherapy of the issues pertinent to Mr. Yee at this stage of his treatment. It was also helpful that Mr. Yee knew of Dr. Tam's reputation as an authority in his field. Dr. Tam used his reputation to help establish an ethnic paternal transference, which made it easier to treat Mr. Yee and achieve a successful outcome.

Dr. Tam not only recognized Mr. Yee's need to be directed by a strong authority figure but also knew that Mr. Yee could not be expected to directly confront his boss. To Mr. Yee, such confrontation would only increase his loss of face. Dr. Tam also knew, from information obtained from Dr. Jones, that the boss had no idea that he had hurt Mr. Yee's feelings in any way. As a labor supervisor, the boss was unlikely to understand Mr. Yee's great sensitivity about "face." Therefore, Dr. Tam chose not to insist on Mr. Yee's return to work. Instead, he used his authority status to direct Mr. Yee in other areas of his life, including medication compliance, health behaviors, interactions with his wife and children, and even interactions with Dr. Tam. In this way, Dr. Tam did not force Mr. Yee to lose more face, but pushed him toward culturally acceptable, psychologically healthy behaviors. This approach worked, and, in fact, as Mr. Yee improved and got mentally stronger, he went back to work.

However, even Dr. Tam, after completing a significant part of the therapy through its middle stage, could not tolerate the patient's noncompliance and residual dependency and had to refer the patient back to Dr. Chang. The medical-psychiatric management of the patient by Dr. Chang at this latter stage of treatment satisfied the need of this patient.

Cultural Influences on Two Key Issues: Dependency and Somatization

Among all the problems that this patient manifested, two cardinal themes stand out: the issues of dependency and somatization. These are rather common issues presented by patients of certain cultural backgrounds, including Asian cultures, and they deserve special consideration and understanding for proper therapeutic management.

Independence and autonomy are desirable and expected of an adult in contemporary American culture. This value affects the philosophical orientation of the psychotherapist. In contrast, *dependence* is generally acceptable, if not conceived of as a virtue, in many other cultures. This was documented by Doi (1973), whose work clarified how dependency is a core issue necessary to understanding ordinary Japanese behavior. He described "blurred ego boundaries" between self and significant others, creating a sense of group rather than individual identity.

T.Y. Lin (1986) described Chinese ideals as being anchored in harmony and synchrony. Chinese culture emphasizes a unitary concept of the mind-body relationship, in contrast to Western culture, where mind and body are separate and dichotomized. One can speculate that this is the origin of the acceptance of somatization common to Asian cultures. Lin goes on to contrast Chinese and Western cultures. Describing the latter, he stated, "The relationship between the Western person with others and the outside world is characterized by open assertiveness and competition" (p. 686).

The dependency needs and behavior manifested by Mr. Yee were excessive, even for the culturally permitted range for Chinese. He regressed into the formal relation he had had in his early childhood with his primary caretaker, his older sister. This was a rather deeply seated complex that resurfaced at the time of crisis. It was not readily resolved by cognitive interpretation. Improvement from this pathological dependency was achieved only through benevolent tolerance and emotional gratification. It was a particular challenge, not only for the independence-oriented (Western) Dr. Jones but also for the dependency-tolerant (Asian) therapists Drs. Chang and Tam.

Another striking characteristic of Mr. Yee's was his excessive concern about his body-health, with multiple somatic complaints throughout the course of his illness. Such hypochondriacal tendencies are commonly observed among patients of diverse ethnic-cultural backgrounds, but they are more prominent among some Asian patients, whose therapy may be particularly difficult for the Western therapist to handle. The nature of somatic complaints among psychiatric patients needs dynamic understanding with cultural sensitivity (Tseng 1975). Somatization may be comprehended as a culturally sanctioned manner of presenting complaints to the doctor, but there may be psychodynamic meaning behind it. It needs to be allowed, understood, and managed properly, including through psychologically gratifying the patient's needs rather than merely relying on intellectual interpretation. The patient's need to somatize can be rechanneled into a discussion of psychological issues with a balanced somatopsychological orientation.

Noncompliance With Medication

The psychology of prescribing medication includes the matter of compliance and an often unspoken contractual agreement between therapist and patient. It is generally expected in modern (Western) medical practice that a patient is to take medication regularly as prescribed. If, for some reason, the patient does not wish to take the medicine prescribed, it is understood that the patient will discuss this with the physician. It is also understood that the patient will see only one primary physician, and not others, except by referral.

This pattern of medical practice is not necessarily understood or appreciated by a patient from another culture. Help-seeking behaviors are very much shaped and molded by cultural custom. For instance, a Chinese patient may believe he has the right to see as many physicians as he chooses. If he is not satisfied by one physician, he can shop around and see others, either alternatively or simultaneously. He also may feel no obligation to seek help solely from one therapist, and may see no need to tell one therapist about the other. It may even be considered impolite to do so.

Also, the patient assumes his or her own right to decide to take or to discontinue medication, based on his or her own judgment, without necessarily obtaining consent from or even telling the physician about it. However, such behavior will naturally be interpreted by the doctor as "noncompliance." This happened in the case of Mr. Yee. The Western-trained Dr. Tam reacted quite strongly to Mr. Yee's noncompliance, even though his own cultural background would have supposedly enabled him to better understand and tolerate such behavior.

References

Doi T: The Anatomy of Dependence: The Key Analysis of Japanese Behavior. Tokyo, Kodansha International, 1973

Lin TY: Multiculturalism and Canadian psychiatry: opportunities and challenges. Can J Psychiatry 31:681–689, 1986

Tseng WS: The nature of somatic complaint among psychiatric patients: the Chinese case. Compr Psychiatry 16:237–245, 1975

PART 3

Special Issues in Therapy

CHAPTER 7

Lessons From Folk Healing Practices

Richard J. Castillo, Ph.D.

Until quite recently, scientific medicine has been hostile to folk and faith healers. From the perspective of biomedical practice, healers who use various types of folk remedies, nonmedical approaches, and religious methods in their healing practices are engaging in worthless superstition and occultism and may be exploiting or even harming vulnerable patients. Although there are certainly unscrupulous healers whose practice is to financially exploit patients, and other healers who use potentially hazardous methods, recently, a change in attitude toward folk healing practices has been evident within the field of scientific medicine. This is exemplified by the creation of an Office of Alternative Medicine within the National Institutes of Health, traditionally a bastion of scientific conservatism. This change in attitude has been motivated to a significant extent by the wide acceptance and use of folk healing methods by the general public.

Every year, Americans spend an estimated $30 billion for services provided by alternative therapists and faith healers (Wallis 1996). Most of this cost is not yet covered by insurance, but patients are willing to pay for these folk healing treatments out of their own pockets. The obvious question is, What are patients receiving from folk healers, that they experience as therapeutic, that they are not receiving from medical practitioners?

No one would argue that any folk healing method is an adequate substitute for medical care. However, the therapeutic value of folk healing practices, for at least some patients, has been found in many studies (Castillo 1991a, 1991b; Csordas 1983; Frank 1974, 1975; Heinze 1988; Jilek 1993, 1994; Katz 1993; Kleinman 1980; Kortmann 1987; Thong 1993; Trotter and Chavira 1997; Tseng 1976; Zatzick and Johnson 1997). Because these studies were done in the field, they generally were not rigorously controlled. Nevertheless, there is enough evidence to conclude that there are lessons to be learned from folk healing practices that can be applied in modern medical practice and culturally appropriate psychotherapy. Besides treatments that directly affect the body, folk healing methods provide opportunities for cognitive restructuring that can sometimes lead to alleviation of emotional distress, potentially affecting both bodily and mental health.

Basic Concepts and Terms

In understanding the mechanisms of folk healing methods, it is helpful to begin with the anthropological concepts of illness, disease, healing, and curing, all of which have specialized meanings. The term *illness* refers to the subjective experience of the patient. It is the subjective experience of being sick, including the experience of physical dysfunction, emotional distress, help seeking, side effects of treatment, social stigma, explanations of causes, diagnosis, prognosis, and personal consequences in family life and occupation (Kleinman 1988).

In contrast, the term *disease* refers to the diagnosis of the doctor or folk healer. It is the clinician's definition of the patient's problem, always taken from the paradigm of disease in which the clinician was trained. For example, a medical doctor is trained to diagnose biological diseases, a psychoanalyst is trained to diagnose psychodynamic problems, and a folk healer might be trained to diagnose such things as an imbalance in vital energy, demonic possession, soul loss, neglect of ancestral spirits, breach of taboo, or witchcraft. In each case, the clinician's diagnosis is the "disease." In medical anthropology, both the clinician's diagnosis and the patient's subjective illness experience are cognitive constructions based on cultural schemas.

The distinction between illness and disease in anthropology is central to the concept of *clinical reality*. Clinical reality—the cognitive construction of reality in the clinical setting—is created by the clinician and the patient within a clinical context, employing their learned cultural schemas regarding illness and disease. Culture affects the construction of clinical reality in five ways:

1. *Culture-based subjective experience.* In a culture that includes the possibility of spirit possession, patients can subjectively experience themselves as being possessed by demons, ghosts, gods, and other spirits.
2. *Culture-based idioms of distress.* Idioms of distress are the ways patients behave to express that they are ill. These include overt pathological behaviors, seeking of clinical care, mannerisms, figures of speech, and cognitively emphasizing certain symptoms while ignoring others. An example of an idiom of distress would be a person's behaving as if he or she were possessed by a demon in a culture that includes this possibility.
3. *Indigenous clinicians assess and diagnose problems in ways that are consistent with the local culture (i.e., culture-based diagnosis).* In a culture that includes the possibility of spirit possession, a folk healer might diagnose possession by ghosts or demons. If the patient and the clinician are from the same culture, they will usually agree on the nature of the illness and its cause. In this way, a culture-based clinical reality can construct diseases that are experienced subjectively by patients and confirmed objectively by indigenous healers.
4. *The appropriate treatment for an illness is defined by the culture-based clinical reality (i.e., culture-based treatment).* For example, the culture-based treatment for a patient possessed by demons could be an exorcism ritual.
5. *Outcomes occur because an illness has been cognitively constructed and treated in a particular cultural fashion (i.e., culture-based outcome).* For example, the outcome for spirit possession when the patient is treated with appropriate folk healing can be good, with complete remission of symptoms (Jilek 1993; Thong 1993).

Special problems in constructing a clinical reality occur if the patient and the clinician come from different cultural backgrounds. If their cultures are different, the illness experienced by the patient is not likely to be the same as the disease diagnosed by the clinician. Because clinicians are trained to treat the diseases defined by their own cultural reality or professional paradigm, the prescribed treatments always match the diagnosed diseases. Treating the diagnosed disease while ignoring the patient's illness (subjective experience) has been described by Kleinman (1988) as *curing*. In contrast, treating the patient's illness is defined as *healing*. Ignoring the patient's illness and only treating the diagnosed disease can result in medical noncompliance and poor outcome (Singh 1985). Clinicians need to be aware of both illness and disease so that they can administer both curing and healing.

A folk healer is someone who treats the patient's subjective experience of illness instead of a disease as recognized by biomedicine. In contrast, physicians tend to practice curing (treating diseases as defined by biomedicine) rather than healing (treating the subjective illnesses of patients). Therefore, in order to receive treatment for their illnesses (healing), patients go to folk healers instead of medical practitioners. Illnesses that are most effectively treated by folk healing are those related to or affected by emotional distress, such as anxiety, depression, somatization, and dissociation.

Coherence in Healing

The effectiveness of folk healing is directly related to its ability to relieve emotional distress in the patient. Much of what constitutes an experience of emotional distress is made up of cognitive constructions. Aaron Antonovsky (1979) formulated the concept of *coherence* in healing. The connection between cognition and emotional distress is where the concept of coherence becomes central to folk healing. With coherence, a patient has the cognition that one's internal and external environments are predictable and reasonably under control. By gaining coherence, the ill person gains hope and thereby avoids hopelessness. Coherence comprises three components: comprehensibility, manageability, and meaningfulness.

Comprehensibility

Comprehensibility refers to a sense of order: the ill person can understand the source of the illness, the mechanism of illness, and its effects on the body and his or her life. The illness no longer is unknown, but is known and understood. This is very important, because there are fewer things more distressing than the unknown. The unknown can take on any proportions or catastrophic dimensions in the mind of the patient. This kind of cognition can produce highly distressful emotions, thus potentially exacerbating any preexisting emotional or physical disturbance. For this reason, it is very important to provide comprehensibility to a patient. By providing comprehensibility, emotional distress is decreased; patients gain a sense of order in their world and are not faced with the unknown.

Providing comprehensibility is probably one of the main reasons folk healers sometimes get good clinical results. Folk healers know that they need to provide *healing* for the patient's emotions. The explanations of the mechanism of illness—soul loss, soul theft, spirit attack, sin, object intrusion, sorcery, imbalance in vital energy, and so on—may seem absurd from the perspective of biomedicine. However, it is not necessary for these explanations to be true in any absolute sense. They are still capable of providing comprehensibility within a particular clinical reality, and thereby alleviate the patient's emotional distress. The most powerful source of comprehensibility will likely come from the patient's own explanatory model of illness. Therefore, careful assessment of a patient's explanatory model of illness can be very important in applying cultural knowledge to therapy.

Manageability

The second component of coherence in folk healing is *manageability*, a cognition of control or competence to meet the demands of the illness. Just knowing that the situation is not out of control is itself therapeutic. An illness out of control can be extremely distressing, evoking emotions of anxiety, hopelessness, and helplessness and thereby exacerbating illness. By providing manageability, the folk healer provides the patient with the sense that the illness can be handled; there is an effective treatment for it, and perhaps even a cure. Just by having a sense of manageability, the patient can feel better.

The folk treatment methods used to provide manageability can include the manipulation of various types of ritual objects (e.g., drums, rattles, crystals, oils, chants, prayers, sacrificial animals, healing images, spiritual beings) that may appear to be superstitious nonsense from a biomedical perspective. However, all are capable of providing manageability to a given patient in a particular culture-based clinical reality. The type of treatment that will be most effective in providing the symbolic power of manageability, of course, depends on the cultural identity and explanatory model of illness of the patient.

Meaningfulness

The third component of coherence in folk healing, *meaningfulness*, refers to a sense of *purpose* to the illness experience. Meaningfulness is commonly found in various forms of religious folk healing. Religion is capable of providing a moral reason for illness or a religious value in the illness.

Within biomedicine, diseases do not possess meaning in any moral or religious sense or in a way that provides positive value to the patient. Meaningfulness provides a possible mechanism of healing that could be useful for some patients. In a religious clinical reality, illness can result from a breach of taboo, neglect of ancestral spirits, immoral behavior, witchcraft, demonic influence, and so on. By reversing the breach of taboo, appeasing the ancestors, restricting the immoral behavior, removing demonic influence, or ritually purifying the patient, the reasons for the illness can be removed, thus alleviating emotional distress and, perhaps, relieving symptoms. Similarly, by giving the experience of suffering associated with the illness some beneficial religious value, the emotional distress associated with the illness can be relieved, and this also can potentially reduce symptoms.

Folk healers also frequently use religious symbolism to provide opportunities for healing or restructuring social relations. In traditional societies, folk healing almost always involves the patient's family, kin group, or village. Therapy is a collective process in which family and community members can take an active part in defining the nature of the problem, as well as its treatment. A collective therapeutic alliance is thus formed among the folk healer, patient, family, and community that can result in a strengthening of group cohesion or a restructuring of group dynamics. In some cases, there is active social engineering. This can be very important in the alleviation of social stress that could be causing symptoms in some patients (Jilek 1993). In most cases, there is a culture congeniality in which the patient and family have their spiritual and social values reinforced through the manipulation of religious and other culturally validated symbols.

Symbolic Healing

Folk healing practices frequently involve the cognitive restructuring of meaning in the mind of the patient to reduce emotional distress and alleviate symptoms. This process involves what Jerome Frank (1975) has termed the "expectant faith effect," namely, the perceived effectiveness of the healer's methods in the mind of the patient. The more effective the treatment is expected to be, the more effective it will be in practice.

This effectiveness is sometimes facilitated by the creation of a *charismatic relationship* between the healer and the patient. If the healer is perceived as possessing or using spiritual or supernatural power, the treatments are likely to evoke a stronger expectant faith effect in the patient. However, a charismatic relationship is quite different from the therapist-client relationship in Western psychotherapy. In the West (particularly the United States), individuation, self-actualization, and personal independence are generally seen as primary values and desirable goals in life and in psychotherapy. Excessive dependency may be seen as a sign of morbidity and become the focus of treatment. Empowering the patient and promoting personal independence are generally seen as desirable goals in Western psychotherapy.

In contrast, many non-Western cultures are collectivist in nature, emphasizing family and personal relationships built on fundamental premises of interdependency, inequality, and subordination to family and religious authority (Castillo 1997). In a collectivist environment, the ideal of emotional maturity may be seen as a satisfying and continuous dependency relationship. The Western psychotherapeutic terms of *transference* and *countertransference* do not adequately express the degree of emotional involvement that may be expected in the folk healer–patient relationship.

The expectant faith effect has been defined in medical anthropology as *symbolic healing* (Dow 1986). Symbolic healing refers to the use of *healing symbols* (i.e., treatments, ritual objects, and placebos) used in healing practices. The folk healer engaged in symbolic healing isolates part of the patient's set of cultural schemas relevant to the illness and interprets the problem in terms of a negotiated clinical reality. In the therapeutic process, symbols are formed that become intellectually and emotionally charged for the patient. Healing symbols can be any treatments, ritual objects, or actions performed by the healer that facilitate the patient's transformation of subjectively experienced reality and alleviation of emotional distress.

Healing symbols can have both *instrumental* (direct physical effect) and purely *symbolic* (psychological) value. Examples of healing symbols include surgery, various medical procedures, medications, radiation treatment, herbal remedies, massage or healing touch, prayer, meditation, rituals of reconciliation, penance for sin, various ritual objects, specialized diets, exercise, visualization, chanting, proverbs, scriptures, and so on. If the patient accepts the healer's explanation as a valid model of his or her illness, then by skillful manipulation of the healing symbols, the patient's emotions and illness can be therapeutically altered. Dow (1986), following Ehrenwald, refers to this alteration as the "existential shift," that is, a change in the patient's experienced reality that creates new opportunities for psychological adaptation. The manipulation of symbols is greatly facilitated if both healer and patient understand, on the basis of the same set of cultural schemas, the meaning of healing symbols.

In the use of healing symbols with purely symbolic value, it is theorized that therapeutic alterations in physiology are accomplished by alleviating emotional distress. Alterations in emotions affect the nervous, endocrine, and immune systems. Thus, alleviating emotional distress is thought to indirectly affect biological disease processes (Ader et al. 1991; Dow 1986; Holland and Rowland 1989; Lerner 1994).

Folk Healing Practices in Different Cultures

Yogic Healing for *Dhat* Syndrome in India

Dhat syndrome in India is a culture-bound syndrome related to the fear of excessive "semen loss." The traditional Hindu conception of the body includes seven types of *dhatus* (essential elements), of which semen is considered the most important. It is thought that the *dhatus* determine bodily immunity or susceptibility to disease. Thus, the loss of semen is thought to lead to physical and mental weakness and susceptibility to disease, and excessive masturbation and sexual intercourse are thought to produce mental and physical illness. The most common symptoms of *dhat* syndrome are fatigue, weakness, body aches, severe headaches, depressed mood, various anxiety symptoms, loss of appetite, insomnia, heart palpitations, and suicidal feelings (Singh 1985).

Castillo (1991a) reported a case of *dhat* syndrome in a 38-year-old male clothing merchant in Bihar, India. The patient explained the origin of his symptoms:

> Now I can tell you one thing, during my high school days I was—well—I will put all the facts very openly before you. I was in the acute habit of masturbation. And this habit of masturbation had me very weak and feeble. Because, all the time I used to indulge in sexual feelings—thinking about that. Always, you can say, daydreaming. So I used to be lost in daydreaming—doing masturbation. *Extremely.* So all this made me very weak, much more weak mentally than physically. And I connect the causes of the mental illness with that.

As is shown in this case, the symptoms were related to the patient's perceived excessive loss of semen. Because his symptoms later remitted when he was able to restrict sexual activity, it is clear that the illness was intimately related to elements of Hindu cultural beliefs concerning sexuality, illness, and healing, which served as models for subjective experience. Thus, cultural symbols were structuring the clinical reality of the illness and experience of healing.

The patient's illness was successfully treated by a Hindu folk healer, who prescribed yoga meditation and reduction in sexual activity. It was thought by the healer that emotional detachment from sexual desire was necessary for the patient to successfully restrict sexual activity. That detachment could be acquired only through yoga meditation. Within the Hindu yoga belief system, emotional detachment is achieved by developing a division in consciousness (dissociation). Yogis use meditation and the resulting dissociation to psychologically transcend problems in life as well as emotional distress and anxiety. They create, through meditation, a secondary, "observing" self that is removed from the problems and emotional distress present in the life of the primary self. Thus, yogic healing can be considered a form of Hindu folk psychotherapy (Castillo 1991a, 1991b).

The patient referred to his "observing" self created through meditation as "the Spectator":

> Now, I will tell you how I did correct it—how I got rid of it. This Spectator in me helped me a lot in this context. I used to be afraid that I had not locked my shop properly. I would return ten or fifteen times to check it. Now, whenever I would have this problem I would shut my eyes and concentrate on that Spectator mind, that is, higher level of mind. And I would confirm from him that I had locked it well. And there was a type of autosuggestion from my higher mind to my shaky mind, "You don't behave like that, you have locked it properly." Then my shakiness and sense of insecurity and all these things would go, and it would be all right. This type of practice, getting help from the Spectator mind, from the higher level of mind, was very helpful in getting my lower mind disciplined and peaceful. So this type of autosuggestion has worked a lot in my life. And not only this, while doing meditation, at the end of meditation I would concentrate on my Spectator mind and will pass on autosuggestions that "throughout this day, I will be normal. I will think and react normally." Through these autosuggestions the reactions I had would be just like a normal man. So this Spectator mind has been of great use to me in eliminating my mental problems.
>
> Now, I was facing the problem of sleeplessness. For a long time I did not sleep continuously for 2 hours, or even for 1 hour. So that sleeplessness was also there. To help this I used to meditate very intensively. When I was in meditation, I would be all right. I would feel all right. After meditation there were no symptoms, no heart palpitations, no unnecessary anxiety. And that effect of meditation would continue for some hours, but again, after that, I would be the victim of all those things. I can say that this meditation was a great support to me. Because, the more I would meditate, the greater would be the intensity of that Spectator, the greater would be the grip of that Spectator on my mental condition. So that way, meditation helped me a lot. When I have that Spectator there is no anxiety—nothing— nothing. I feel very much elevated. I feel that I am a great Soul. I feel I could do anything in this world. No fear—nothing.

The most common clinical diagnosis made by Western-trained psychiatrists in India for patients with *dhat* syndrome is major depression (Singh 1985). However, the outcome for these patients when treated exclusively with antidepressants is poor, because pharmacotherapy in and of itself does not address their subjective experience of illness. As Singh (1985, p. 122) states:

> Follow up of these patients is very poor, majority (64 percent) did not come again after the first visit and hence the response to anti-depressant treatment could not be assessed. It is probably that these patients were not satisfied with our explanation that seminal loss was not harmful but that their symptoms were due to their excessive worrying about this for which we would prescribe them the treatment. On the contrary it seems extremely naive to believe that after telling a patient that he is not suffering from the illness for which he has come, we should expect him to take our treatment for an illness which he does not believe even exists.

Thus, the successful treatment of *dhat* syndrome is more likely to be achieved if the culture-based illness experience of the patient is made the focus of treatment. This may require the use of folk healing methods such as yoga meditation.

Religious Healing Among American Charismatic Christians

Thomas Csordas (1983) and Meredith McGuire (1988) have described three types of religious folk healing methods used by some charismatic Christian healers in the United States: spiritual healing, healing of memories, and deliverance. *Spiritual healing* is conceptualized by the Christian healers as God healing a soul that has been injured by sin. *Healing of memories* is treatment for traumatic memories that may be troubling a person, even after that person has received the Holy Spirit. *Deliverance* is treatment characterized by freeing a person from the adverse effects of demons or evil spirits. In this case, a distinction is made between *oppression,* in which the effect of a demon is experienced in some limited aspect of a person's life, and *possession,* in which a demon takes over complete control of a person. Oppression by a demon usually takes the form of sinful behavior, such as lust, masturbation, adultery, and so on. Possession by a demon is essentially the charismatic Christian equivalent of spirit possession illnesses observed in various parts of the premodern world. Deliverance can be described as the charismatic Christian version of exorcism. The offending demon is contacted, addressed by name, and commanded to depart in the name of Jesus Christ.

The healing-of-memories method is somewhat different from deliverance and illustrates clearly the structure of symbolic healing. In healing of memories, the individual's entire life is prayed for in chronological stages, from conception to the present. Special attention is paid to any events or relationships that caused the individual emotional pain or trauma. The individual is usually asked to visualize the painful incident but to alter the original memory by visualizing Jesus there at the person's side, more or less guiding the person through that painful event. The meaning of the event is thus altered. The goal is to have the patient accept that Jesus was there all the time and wanted the person to go through that difficult time in order to bring the person closer to Him. Thus, the meaning of the event is altered. This process is done for all stressful events, in effect, "walking Jesus through" the person's life, thus altering the meaning of all those events and, therefore, the emotions associated with them (i.e., providing meaningfulness). By placing Jesus in those traumatic or stressful events, the events are given a beneficial meaning and a purpose they did not previously possess. Therefore, the feelings of sadness, shame, guilt, horror, anger, resentment, fear, helplessness, and so on, that were previously associated with those memories are no longer applicable and can be replaced by feelings of love, gratitude, and happiness. This can have immediate and significant healing effects on the patient. It is not necessary for any of this to be true in any absolute sense; it is only necessary for it to be symbolically powerful for the patient.

Cognitive processes are central to the healing of emotional distress. Cultural schemas can carry within them sources of both emotional distress and emotional healing. It is the job of the clinician to discover what these sources are for each patient and to use them to provide coherence in therapy. It is therefore extremely important to carefully assess all patients, including their cultural schemas and explanatory models, and to use that information in therapy.

Shamanic Healing of Spirit Possession in South Asia

In South Asian cultural schemas, particularly in the rural areas, it is generally accepted that ghosts and demons may possess persons and cause illness and antisocial behavior. It is also generally accepted that gods and goddesses may possess persons. In the latter case, the possession is a spiritual gift and an expression of the power of the deity. It is also generally accepted that gods have power over ghosts and demons; gods may punish ghosts and demons and order them to depart. Sometimes, elaborate rituals, in which the shaman is possessed by a succession of increasingly powerful gods with very high status in the spiritual hierarchy, are necessary in order to banish a particularly difficult demon (e.g., McDaniel 1989; Obeyesekere 1977, 1981).

In the treatment of demonic possession by symbolic healing, the shaman usually induces a state of trance in the patient, if he or she is not already in an active state of possession. The shaman can thereby converse directly with the possessing demon and determine its identity, the reasons it is possessing the victim, and what it wants in exchange for its departure. Negotiations between the shaman and the demon are then begun. Frequently, the demon refuses to leave, and the shaman must threaten the demon with supernatural harm from his own spiritual powers. Usually the shaman will have one or more gods that he can call on in a state of trance to possess him (take control of his body) and do battle with the demons possessing the patient. The healing rituals are primarily aimed at establishing, negotiating, and manipulating the symbolic relations between the shaman's god and the patient's demon.

In the shamanic treatment of demonic possession in South Asia, the healer and patient share a common set of cultural schemas (Dow's step 1; see Dow 1986). The shaman then negotiates a clinical reality between himself and the possessed person, taken from the cultural schemas (step 2). This defines the nature of the participants for the ensuing rituals and the relative status of the parties. That is, the shaman, in conjunction with the patient, diagnoses a particular type of demonic possession that requires a particular type of healing ritual.

The shaman then involves the patient's intellect and emotions with healing symbols (step 3). In South Asia, the symbols, taken from the cultural schemas, are typically recited sacred verses (mantras) or the presence of a particular deity who possesses the shaman (highlighted by appropriate costuming and props) and who is acknowledged within the meaning system to have the power to banish demons. Other ritual objects, such as amulets or charmed strings tied around the patient's wrist or neck, may also be used. In addition, a cutting of the patient's hair may be ritually consigned to some sort of sacred container (e.g., a cloth or clay pot) and removed from the premises or ritually burned, symbolizing removal of the spirit. Various offerings and gifts to the spirit may also serve the purpose of healing symbols.

By skillful manipulation of these healing symbols, the shaman transforms the meaning of the demon's existential status, effectively altering the subjective experience of the patient (step 4). It must be noted that the patient is usually in a trance and, therefore, highly susceptible to hypnotic suggestion. The shaman uses this heightened suggestibility to persuade, cajole, and threaten the demon into leaving, thus healing the patient.

Shamanic Healing of "Spirit Loss" in Nepal

One of the most common forms of illness among the Yolmo Sherpa people of Nepal is a malady that can be translated as "spirit loss." The Yolmo believe that one's spirit can be caused to leave the body by being suddenly frightened or emotionally traumatized. The spirit then wanders around the country-side, prey to ghosts, demons, and witches. When this happens, the individual experiences extreme fatigue, lacks the will for activity, and does not care to eat, talk, work, or socialize. Insomnia and other symptoms may also be present (Des Jarlais et al. 1995). From the perspective of modern psychiatry, the patient appears to be suffering from major depression.

When a Yolmo suffers from spirit loss, a shaman is brought in to per-form an all-night healing ritual, in which he or she recites sacred chants, is possessed by deities who inform about the causes of the patient's illness, and manipulates other symbolic objects. Toward the end of the healing ritual, the shaman performs a "spirit-hooking" ceremony, in which his or her own spir-it leaves his or her body and flies out like a bird to search for the patient's lost spirit. Upon locating the lost spirit, the shaman "hooks" it and returns with it to the patient's house, where he or she deposits the spirit into several foods set before the patient. By eating from each of these foods, the patient recovers his or her spirit and is healed of the symptoms (Desjarlais et al. 1995).

Tribal Healing of Alcoholism Among Native Americans

Alcoholics Anonymous (AA) groups, developed in a Western cultural frame-work, have not generally been successful among North American Indian populations (Heath 1983). This lack of success is to be expected, because the healing symbols used in the AA healing ceremonies are not consistent with Native American culture. Healing systems consistent with Native American culture would have more symbolic healing power. Therefore, in recent de-cades, many Indian groups have revived the sweat lodge ceremony for the healing of alcoholism (Hall 1986).

Hot rocks are placed in the center of the sweat lodge and sprinkled with water to release steam. In the small enclosed space, the steam produces pro-fuse sweating in participants, who sit in a circle facing the center. Beyond the instrumental therapeutic effects of the sweating, the ceremony uses symbol-ic objects manipulated by a spiritual leader to alter the cognitions and emo-tions of the participants. The ceremony itself and the objects used within it are symbols of the revival of the American Indian culture and the removal of the harmful effects of the dominant white culture. The ceremony is experienced as a purification from the pollution of white culture and the effects of alcohol, which are seen as a manifestation of white cultural pollution. The ceremonies are designed to help the individuals strengthen their Indian personal and group identities; relieve depression related to cultural alienation, relative deprivation, and ethnic identity confusion; and create a new, healthy way of life for the individual and the group (Jilek 1994).

This transformation is achieved in a ritualized symbolic death of the old polluted self and the rebirth of a new, strong, purified Indian self. The sociocentric bonds of traditional Indian culture are renewed and strengthened in the ceremony, and individuals receive the emotional support of group identity and escape the alienation of the egocentric white culture. This creates new social networks, alters negative social relationships, and allows healed individuals to take on new social roles. The sick role of the alcoholic is exchanged for the prestigious role of the supernaturally purified traditional Indian identity (Jilek 1994). This use of culturally validated symbolic healing and group reinforcement of the new healthy identity is more effective in this sociocultural context for the treatment of alcoholism than the typical Western Alcoholic Anonymous healing method.

Shamanic Healing in a Psychiatric Hospital in Bali

Religion is all-pervasive in Balinese culture. Deities and spirits are encountered everywhere by the Balinese people, collectively constructed and maintained by the Balinese cultural schemas. In this culture, all these cognitively created supernatural entities are capable of possessing a person and causing various illnesses. Likewise, Balinese sorcerers can cause illness by manipulating various minor spirits and, through the technique of "object intrusion," are believed to cause illness by magically implanting a harmful object in a victim. Furthermore, the Balinese are highly aware of geographical orientation in relation to the holy mountain at the center of the island. Without constant awareness of this geographical direction, the Balinese will experience *paling*, a disoriented, confused state in which they are unable to function.

Mental illness is called *buduh* in Bali and has indigenous symptoms: *inguh, pusing, paling,* and *lengeh,* being dizzy, confused, or disoriented; *ngamuk,* running amok; *bengong* and *samun,* being apathetic or dazed; *ngumikmik,* raving, being incoherent, or talking to oneself; *nyeh,* being anxious, frightened, or excessively timid; *malumbar,* running away and resisting restraint; and *ngumbang,* wandering aimlessly. The causes of these symptoms are indigenously attributed to inherited factors, possession by spirits and gods, ancestral or divine curses, and sorcery (Connor 1979, cited in Thong 1993).

Thong (1993), a psychiatrist, reported how he developed a Balinese cultural approach in clinical assessment and treatment in the state mental hospital, using shamanic healing methods. His clinical results were impressive. First, he organized his hospital and staff into a *banjar*, the smallest and most basic unit of social organization in Bali next to the family. The *banjar* consists of 500–1,500 people and confers a highly important social identity and spiritual connection on its members. Each banjar has its own temple, which serves as a seat for the *banjar*'s god and a location for religious festivals. To organize a *banjar*, Dr. Thong and his staff had to build a temple on the hospital grounds and perform religious rituals there. Through this, the temple became the seat of Djero Gede, a powerful Balinese god who could heal the sick. This spiritual power became an important part of Thong's symbolic arsenal for dealing with mental disorders. Emotional distress was relieved by the symbolic power of the god and the temple. Some patients felt better just by walking onto the grounds of the hospital.

Next, Dr. Thong looked at the architecture of the hospital. He discovered that, because hospitals had been designed by Dutch colonials many years earlier, none of them took into account the sacred geography of Bali. Balinese are forbidden to sleep with their heads in certain directions. If this rule is disobeyed, it can cause anxiety and confusion. Yet, hospitals in Bali, built on a Western model of a large hall with two rows of beds on either side, took no notice of this part of Balinese culture. Beds pointed in the wrong direction were likely to evoke anxiety in the patients, worsening their mental disorders.

To avoid the culturally inappropriate architecture of the hospital, Thong built what he called the "Family Ward." This ward was a complex of four compounds, built in traditional Balinese style, each capable of housing one patient and his or her family. In the Family Ward, patients received the usual psychiatric medications, but the families were allowed to stay with the patients. Also, the hospital staff spent much more time with the patients and families than in the usual hospital setting, involving them in therapy and discussing their personal and family problems. In addition, if the patient or family requested it, a Balinese folk healer (*balian*) was brought in to treat the patient. Thong even went so far as to make a *balian* a regular part of the staff. He found the *balian* to be very competent in treating *bebainan* (illness caused by sorcery), spirit possession, psychotic episodes, family disputes, and "bad luck," as well as muscular problems, bone fractures, and mild fevers.

Dr. Thong and the *balians* treated the *illnesses* of their Balinese patients, as well as their diseases. This approach was vital to optimal outcome for each patient. As Thong (1993) stated, "The Balinese patient will not rest until he or she has seen a healer who will agree to treat the supernatural cause that brought about the ailment" (p. 114). Thus, Thong found that when the subjective illness as constructed by the patient's cultural schemas was not treated, outcome was poor.

During the 1 year that the Family Ward was in operation, 14 patients were treated there. Nine were diagnosed with a chronic mental illness (7 with schizophrenia, 1 with endogenous depression, and 1 with substance use disorder). Of the 9 chronic patients, 7 recovered and 2 remained hospitalized. The 7 who recovered spent an average of 40 days in the Family Ward and were released. Dr. Thong attributed the high rate of recovery to the fact that they were treated in the Family Ward, in a more traditional Balinese fashion. Thus, the treatment was a combination of folk healing and modern psychiatry. Similar experiences of successfully treating Balinese patients with folk healing methods were also reported by Suryani and Jensen (1993). Clinicians all over the world can learn from these physicians' cultural sensitivity and their clinical applications of folk healing methods.

In Bali, Thong (1993) prescribed the usual psychiatric medications for his patients, while simultaneously using the patients' own folk models for providing comprehensibility for their illnesses, and obtained very good clinical results. Thus, it is not necessary to educate and convert every patient to a modern scientific model of thinking to provide comprehensibility. Modern psychiatric explanations are not necessarily more comprehensible to any given patient. Indeed, it is much easier and quicker to use the explanatory model that the patient brings to the clinical situation.

New Age Folk Healing in the United States

Zatzick and Johnson (1997) described the practice and clinical results of a New Age folk healer who treats middle-class Americans. New Age folk healing is a heterogeneous mix of therapies, including religious healing, Native American shamanic practices, Eastern meditation techniques, hypnotherapies, psychic and occult healing, self-help groups, and various kinds of massage and physical manipulation therapies. The folk healer studied by Zatzick and Johnson had developed his own brand of therapy called "Self-Acceptance Training," which employed trance induction, guided imagery, and various Native American shamanic techniques, such as drumming, chanting, shamanic journeying to "upper" and "lower" worlds, soul retrieval, "depossession" of offending spirits, use of "power animals," and symbolic dismemberment and reconstruction of the client.

This healer did not treat diseases as recognized by biomedicine; he treated the psychological concomitants of physical disease, psychosomatic ailments, and the psychological effects of traumatic events—that is, the *illness* of the patient. The most prominent factor was "self-acceptance" through cognitive restructuring of negative and destructive self-evaluations stemming from highly stressful and traumatic past events. The healing was accomplished by neutralizing the negative psychological effects of these events.

After inducing a trance in the client, the healer would access negative or traumatic memories in order to reexperience those events. The healer would then begin a methodical process of altering the emotions of the client through a positive reconstruction of the negative events. This was accomplished through the introduction of healing images, such as "power animals," that furnished the client with the spiritual power to overcome the traumatic events. If the clients could become absorbed in this imagery, they experienced a therapeutic reconstruction of past events. Those events were now associated with positive emotions. No attempt was made to forget the past; rather, the past was reconstructed to allow for an alleviation of emotional distress associated with the past. The goal was to replace anxiety and depression with a positive sense of mastery and control. The structure of this healing practice is very similar to the "healing of memories" method used by charismatic Christians (discussed earlier in this chapter) and follows the general pattern of symbolic healing described earlier.

The clinical results of the healer studied by Zatzick and Johnson (1997) were generally positive. Only one of nine clients followed for a year reported any negative effects. (These consisted of occasional flashbacks and anxiety, associated with a shamanic "depossession" ceremony.) The other eight clients reported generally positive results, although only two reported significant and lasting positive change at 1-year follow-up. Others reported less significant or transient positive changes.

Conclusion

Every year, Americans spend an estimated $30 billion for services provided by alternative therapists and faith healers. Even though this cost is usually not covered by insurance, patients go to these healers because their treatments are culturally congruent with patients' beliefs about illness and healing and are thus experienced as therapeutic. Because of the use of culturally validated healing symbols, patients' emotional distress can be therapeutically altered, potentially relieving the subjective experience of symptoms.

Folk healing is the treatment of illness in a manner consistent with a particular folk *clinical reality*. Folk healers treat the patient's subjective experience rather than a disease as recognized by biomedicine. Medical doctors tend to practice *curing* (treating biological diseases) rather than *healing* (treating the subjective experiences of patients). Therefore, in order to receive treatment for their illnesses (healing), patients go to folk healers instead of medical practitioners.

Illnesses that are most effectively treated by folk healing are those related to or affected by emotional distress, such as anxiety, depression, somatization, and dissociation. Alterations in emotions affect the nervous, endocrine, and immune systems. Thus, alleviating emotional distress is thought to indirectly affect biological disease. This avenue of treatment of biological disease through alleviation of emotional distress is something that is only now becoming fully appreciated and utilized in medical practice.

Folk healing uses both *instrumental* and *symbolic* healing methods. The clinical use of healing symbols is greatly facilitated if both healer and patient understand the meaning of healing symbols on the basis of the same set of cultural schemas. Therefore, a careful cultural assessment of the illness experience and explanatory model should be a routine clinical practice. From this cultural assessment of illness, the use of the patient's own healing symbols can be used in psychotherapy for the alleviation of emotional distress.

Adhering to an exclusively biological model of disease and treatment, or conventional psychotherapy in clinical practice, may be offering a clinical reality and treatment modality that some patients find culturally incongruent and inadequate for alleviating their emotional distress. Trying to educate and convert such patients to a modern scientific understanding of illness and treatment would, in effect, be stripping them of their culture. Such a process is extremely difficult to carry out and probably unnecessary for a good clinical outcome. This is especially true for patients from non-Western cultures or those who are extremely religious.

When serious illness strikes, patients tend to fall back on religious beliefs and rituals or other culturally congruent methods for emotional support and healing. Physicians expressing disapproval of folk or religious healing will not dissuade patients from receiving these treatments. If physicians express hostility toward lay understandings of illness and folk treatments, patients will simply withhold information about folk treatments and remedies they are receiving. This can lead to complications if herbal remedies contain pharmacological agents inconsistent with prescribed medications or if folk treatments are dangerous in some way.

In the worst-case scenario, patients may delay receiving needed medical care in favor of folk or religious healing until their conditions become very advanced. If physicians were more open to including patients' lay explanatory models and healing symbols in a negotiated clinical reality, even to the point of including safe and nonexploitative folk methods in the treatment plan, the doctor-patient relationship would be benefited from the greater openness in the patient and trust in the relationship that such a negotiated clinical reality would engender. Physicians could then exercise more control over treatment. This would guarantee that patients receive necessary medical care, while simultaneously taking advantage of the emotional healing value of safe folk methods. Doctors would be better able to protect patients from financial exploitation by unscrupulous folk healers and from dangerous treatments.

References

Ader R, Felton DL, Cohen N (eds): Psychoneuroimmunology, 2nd Edition. San Diego, CA, Academic Press, 1991

Antonovsky A: Health, Stress, and Coping. San Francisco, CA, Jossey-Bass, 1979

Castillo RJ: Culture, trance and mental illness: divided consciousness in South Asia. Unpublished doctoral dissertation, Harvard University, Cambridge, Massachusetts, 1991a

Castillo RJ: Divided consciousness and enlightenment in Hindu yogis. Anthropology of Consciousness 2:1–6, 1991b

Castillo RJ: Culture and Mental Illness: A Client-Centered Approach. Pacific Grove, CA, Brooks/Cole, 1997

Connor L: Corpse abuse and trance in Bali: the cultural mediation of aggression. Mankind 12:104–118, 1979

Csordas TJ: The rhetoric of transformation in ritual healing. Cult Med Psychiatry 7:333–375, 1983

Des Jarlais R, Eisenberg L, Good B, et al: World Mental Health: Problems and Priorities in Low-Income Countries. New York, Oxford University Press, 1995

Dow J: Universal aspects of symbolic healing: a theoretical synthesis. American Anthropologist 88:56–69, 1986

Frank JD: Persuasion and Healing: A Comparative Study of Psychotherapy, 2nd Edition. New York, Schocken Books, 1974

Frank JD: Psychotherapy of bodily disease: an overview. Psychother Psychosom 26:192–202, 1975

Hall R: Alcohol treatment in American Indian populations: an indigenous treatment modality compared with traditional approaches. Ann N Y Acad Sci 472:168–178, 1986

Heath DB: Alcohol use among North American Indians: a cross-cultural survey of patterns and problems, in Research Advances in Alcohol and Drug Problems, Vol 7. Edited by Smart RG, Glazer FB, Israel Y, et al. New York, Plenum, 1983, pp 343–396

Heinze RI: Trance and Healing in Southeast Asia Today. Bangkok, White Lotus, 1988

Holland JC, Rowland JH: Handbook of Psychooncology. New York, Oxford University Press, 1989

Jilek WG: Traditional medicine relevant to psychiatry, in Treatment of Mental Disorders: A Review of Effectiveness. Edited by Sartorius N, de Girolamo G, Andrews G, et al. Washington, DC, American Psychiatric Press, 1993, pp 341–383 (published on behalf of the World Health Organization)

Jilek WG: Traditional healing in the prevention and treatment of alcohol and drug abuse. Transcultural Psychiatric Research Review 31:219–258, 1994

Katz R: The Straight Path: A Story of Healing and Transformation in Fiji. Reading, MA, Addison-Wesley, 1993

Kleinman A: Patients and Healers in the Context of Culture: An Exploration of the Borderland Between Anthropology, Medicine, and Psychiatry. Berkeley, University of California Press, 1980

Kleinman A: The Illness Narratives: Suffering, Healing and the Human Condition. New York, Basic Books, 1988

Kortmann F: Popular, traditional and professional mental health care in Ethiopia. Transcultural Psychiatric Research Review 24:255–274, 1987

Lerner M: Choices in Healing: Integrating the Best of Conventional and Complementary Approaches to Cancer. Cambridge, MA, MIT Press, 1994

McDaniel J: The Madness of the Saints: Ecstatic Religion in Bengal. Chicago, IL, University of Chicago Press, 1989

McGuire MB: Ritual Healing in Suburban America. New Brunswick, NJ, Rutgers University Press, 1988

Obeyesekere G: Psychocultural exegesis of a case of spirit possession in Sri Lanka, in Case Studies in Spirit Possession. Edited by Crapanzano V, Garrison V. New York, Wiley, 1977, pp 235–294

Obeyesekere G: Medusa's Hair: An Essay on Personal Symbols and Religious Experience. Chicago, IL, University of Chicago Press, 1981

Singh G: Dhat syndrome revisited. Indian Journal of Psychiatry 27:119–122, 1985

Suryani LK, Jensen GD: Trance and Possession in Bali. New York, Oxford University Press, 1993

Thong D: A Psychiatrist in Paradise: Treating Mental Illness in Bali. Bangkok, White Lotus, 1993

Trotter RT, Chavira JA: Curanderismo: Mexican American Folk Healing, 2nd Edition. Athens, University of Georgia Press, 1997

Tseng WS: Folk psychotherapy in Taiwan, in Culture-Bound Syndromes, Ethnopsychiatry, and Alternative Therapies. Edited by Lebra WP. Honolulu, University of Hawaii Press, 1976, pp 164–178

Wallis C: Religious healing. Time, June 24, 1996, pp 58–62

Zatzick DF, Johnson FA: Alternative psychotherapeutic practice among middle class Americans, I: case studies and followup. Cult Med Psychiatry 21:53–88, 1997

CHAPTER 8

Therapist-Patient Relations and Ethnic Transference

David M. Bernstein, M.D.

This chapter provides an overview of important considerations in the relationship between patient and therapist from the perspective of culture and ethnicity. When one attempts an analysis of the influence of culture on the "therapeutic dyad" (Comas-Diaz and Jacobsen 1991) by reviewing the literature on the nature of the therapeutic relationship, the complexity of the topic is evident. The literature addresses concerns inherent in this complex relationship. Such concerns include fundamental conceptual constructs regarding the nature of a "healer" and a patient, the explanatory model of illness (Kleinman 1980), and communicative and linguistic aspects of psychotherapy (Comas-Diaz and Griffith 1988; Ridley 1985). Issues concerning the applicability of various psychotherapeutic orientations (e.g., psychoanalytic) across cultures (Kakar 1985; Yi 1995) are also problematic. Dimou (1995) captures the essence of this difficulty for the therapist who struggles to add an awareness of cultural factors to the therapeutic relationship: "We can imagine that many doctors could feel overwhelmed by the burden imposed upon them, when considering the links between illness and culture. They could react by saying: 'Well—what do you expect me to be when I talk to a patient: a philosopher, a psychologist, an anthropologist, a sociologist, a semanticist, a historian of cultures—and a physician?'"

This chapter highlights several key theoretical concepts applied toward an understanding of the therapist-patient relationship, for the broader purpose of offering suggestions and guidance applicable to commonly encountered clinical situations. An area that receives special emphasis is that of cultural transference and countertransference, which, when strictly defined, are grounded in the psychoanalytic paradigm. In this chapter, the definition has been expanded to include other aspects of the therapeutic relationship, such as prejudice. The variance between patient and therapist regarding gender, age, religion, and ethnicity is addressed within the framework of cultural psychiatry. Therapeutic constructs, such as confidentiality, relationship boundaries, and various elements of the "treatment contract," including patient compliance and expected outcome, are also addressed. The chapter concludes by identifying some common issues related to culture in the therapeutic relationship, with suggestions for management.

Case Vignettes

Mr. Goldberg

Mr. Goldberg, a 55-year-old Jewish male, presented to a mental health clinic with a chief complaint that he was experiencing a diminished enjoyment of his work and was worried he was not realizing his full potential. He specifically requested psychodynamic psychotherapy with a Jewish therapist "to explore general philosophical issues relating to achieving my life's goals." Mr. Goldberg was referred to a Jewish psychiatrist for treatment. At the time of the initial assessment, the patient presented as a high-functioning man with a secure job in a mid-level managerial position for an investment banking firm. He reported that he was in a stable marriage and was not having any relationship difficulties at work or at home; he stressed that "the purpose of this therapy should be geared toward personal insight, and not toward resolution of any specific conflict." Mr. Goldberg denied any symptoms consistent with a mood disorder, psychotic disorder, or anxiety disorder. Mental status examination was unremarkable, as was a recent medical examination.

Mr. Goldberg's developmental history included high scholastic achievement that culminated in a master's degree in business administration from an Ivy League school. He related that, despite being raised in an orthodox Jewish household, he never felt particularly religious and he did not practice Judaism. His father, a successful merchant, pushed Mr. Goldberg to become a rabbi, believing this would be a noble use of his intellectual gift. Although he was educated in *Yeshiva* (Jewish religious schools) until graduation from high school, to the great disappointment of his father, Mr. Goldberg insisted on a secular college education. After completing his master's degree, Mr. Goldberg began working for a series of finance-related firms, eventually rising to a middle-management position.

His first contact with mental health treatment was at age 30, when, disappointed that he had not achieved a higher level of job accomplishment, he sought psychiatric assistance for mild depressive symptoms. He was in psychoanalysis for 2 years, which he felt was helpful. He had married a non-Jewish woman when he was 27 and denied any marital problems. The couple had a teenage daughter, who was doing well in college.

When asked why he wanted a Jewish therapist, he responded that he wanted someone with a *Yiddishe kup* (a Jewish head), a common Jewish expression, meaning that Jews think differently from non-Jews. Mr. Goldberg was seen for 20 sessions of psychodynamic psychotherapy with a Jewish psychiatrist. The therapist noted him to be cooperative yet controlling in the sessions, using intellectualization and obsessional thinking as major defense mechanisms. The therapist was struck by Mr. Goldberg's narcissism and the adolescent qualities of his conflicts regarding rebellion against his past, yet insecurity about having chosen the wrong career path, as evidenced by his self-described "mediocre performance at work." He often came to sessions with pages of "important information," such as descriptions of dreams or cinema critiques, which he insisted the therapist review. He also presented the therapist with multiple articles concerning Judaism, which he felt would be interesting for the therapist, and often chided the therapist for his ignorance of the material. His speech during sessions was replete with Yiddish expressions, and he expressed a sense of enjoyment if he had to explain their meaning to the therapist. When the therapist interpreted this behavior as an attempt to devalue the therapist, the patient responded, "You sound just like my Dad. I appreciate all you've done in therapy, which has been tremendously helpful, but isn't it possible that you could learn something from me?" He completed the allotted 20 sessions, which he viewed as a positive experience, and at the time of termination from therapy he reported that he was functioning well at work, without any feelings of inadequacy. He thanked the therapist and stated, "If I need a tune-up in the future, I'll contact you again."

Discussion

Let us examine this vignette on the basis of some concepts regarding the effect of culture on the therapeutic process that will be discussed in this chapter. Mr. Goldberg presented on his own to the therapist. At the time of his presentation, he self-identified the nature of his problem, as well as the desired mode of therapy. He specifically requested a therapist of similar ethnicity, basing his request on the belief that their shared ethnic background would facilitate the therapeutic process. Mr. Goldberg had previous experience with psychoanalytic psychotherapy, a highly specialized mental health treatment, despite the fact that he was highly functional within his society. His therapist identified particular defense mechanisms, and during the therapy a paternal transference developed. During therapy, Mr. Goldberg consistently devalued the therapist, and when confronted by the therapist, he reacted defensively, pointing out that perhaps the therapist could learn from him. Mr. Goldberg's gifts to the therapist were interpreted as homework assignments, through which he attempted to control the therapy.

While this case may appear typical for a Western-oriented therapist trained in psychodynamic therapy, the behavior, beliefs, and nature of treatment may evoke incredulity from a non-Western perspective. For example, had Mr. Goldberg been Japanese, living in Japan, it is unlikely that he would ever have been in mental health treatment while functioning well by societal standards. If he were in therapy, it likely would not be by his own volition. Seeking mental health treatment for purposes of self-enhancement would be viewed as selfish and inappropriate. If he were ill enough to warrant mental health treatment, he would likely have been brought in by his family, who would expect to be included in treatment. The idea of patient confidentiality would be a nonissue, because treatment would not be based on the idea of an exclusive patient-therapist dyadic relationship. Mr. Goldberg would likely assume a passive role and would not specify the background of the therapist or question his credentials either overtly or covertly in session. Gifts from Mr. Goldberg or his family would be expected, and accepted, if deemed reasonable, not interpreted.

The notion of a patient controlling the therapy in any fashion, rather than passively accepting the therapist's diagnosis and treatment, would be unlikely in Japanese culture and viewed as improper patient behavior. Mr. Goldberg would not attempt to devalue or educate the therapist. Rather, if he or his family were unhappy with the treatment, they would either passively accept it during sessions and not implement it when at home (e.g., be noncompliant with medications prescribed) or tactfully end treatment in a nonconfrontational manner. This would allow the therapist to "save face," even if the Goldberg family decided to pursue treatment with a different therapist. The "noncompliance" would not be viewed as a pathological defense mechanism (e.g., acting out or passive-aggressive behavior), because such behavior is culturally sanctioned in a society that values indirect communication.

Mrs. Tran

Mrs. Tran, a 47-year-old Vietnamese woman, presented to the university mental health clinic after being referred by her primary care physician. The physician's consult note indicated that Mrs. Tran received a workup for headaches and abdominal pains, with negative findings. She suspected that Mrs. Tran's symptoms were stress-related. On intake, Mrs. Tran described a vague pattern of headaches and abdominal pain that began shortly after her immigration to the United States nearly 1 year before. She was unemployed and living on public assistance, along with her unemployed husband and 15-year-old son, who was attending a public high school. Mrs. Tran's English was poor, and the Caucasian American male therapist requested a Vietnamese translator. During the next session, Mrs. Tran revealed feeling stress from her relationship with her husband, and she also reported that her son was having problems at school. The therapist requested a couple's session, to which Mrs. Tran and her husband reluctantly agreed.

During the session, the couple described their son as having problems with the police, because he was missing school and associating with a Vietnamese gang in Chinatown. When the therapist attempted to get more history regarding the family, Mr. Tran stated that their son was an orphaned half–African American, half-Vietnamese child, whom the couple had adopted during the war. The therapist, who felt a sense of gratitude and admiration for the couple, was disconcerted when the translator began to chuckle. After the session, the therapist asked the translator about this incident. The translator informed the therapist that no Vietnamese would adopt a mixed-race child, particularly during a war. He suspected that the child was purchased as a teenager from brokers in Vietnam, who sell such children because United States immigration policy allows these children to return to the United States, accompanied by their parents. Such children are thus precious commodities who are purchased by people wishing to immigrate to the United States.

At the next session the therapist, angry that he had been deceived, and outraged that children were treated as a commodity to defraud the United

States government, confronted the couple about this issue. After initially denying it, Mr. Tran eventually admitted that he and his wife had entered the country in this manner. They had purchased phony adoption papers in Vietnam. They were upset that the adolescent child was causing problems with the police, and fearfully asked the therapist if he would notify the Immigration Service and have them all deported. The therapist explained the policy of confidentiality and assured the couple that the Immigration Service would not be notified. The couple did not show up for the next appointment. All attempts to schedule future appointments were fruitless, and the couple was lost to follow-up. The translator was not surprised by this outcome.

Discussion

This case illustrates several important issues in the therapist-patient relationship across cultures. The therapist, recognizing that language would be an impediment to treatment, obtained the assistance of a translator. The translator's seemingly inappropriate response during the session prompted the therapist to use the translator as a cultural expert, whose role was expanded to provide the therapist with insight into contemporary Vietnamese society. The therapist initially experienced feelings of admiration for this seemingly heroic couple, who struggled to help a child of mixed American ancestry, born during a war that has come to represent a tragic failure of American foreign policy. These feelings reflected the therapist's own cognitions and emotions about the Vietnam War. Upon learning the true motivation of the couple, which involved immigration fraud centered around the use of children as commodities, the therapist's feelings changed to anger and outrage. This contrasted sharply with the translator's feeling of amusement that a scam so widely known in the Vietnamese community would have gone undetected by the supposedly sophisticated therapist.

The therapist confronted the couple with this information as part of a larger therapeutic strategy. This confrontation was likely perceived by the couple as a threat to involve the government, which would result in punitive action. This perception was likely grounded in the sociopolitical climate in Vietnam, with which the couple had firsthand experience. Thus, the eventual outcome of this case was unremarkable to the culturally informed translator. Whereas the therapist's main concern was the mental health of the patient, the couple's main concern was the preservation of their immigration status. The therapist attempted to explain the concept of therapist-patient confidentiality, in the hope of maintaining the therapy. The couple, unable to accept this concept, abandoned therapy in order to preserve their precious immigration status.

The Therapeutic Relationship: Literature Review

It is useful to approach an analysis of a relationship as complex as the therapeutic relationship by first examining factors relating to the participants in the relationship. Although, on the surface, it may seem easy to identify the therapist and the patient as central to the therapeutic relationship, a deeper view, from a cultural perspective, raises fundamental identity questions: 1) Who is the therapist, and what makes him or her qualified to fulfill this role; and 2) Who is the patient? Should the therapist define the patient as the individual in the treatment room, or as part of a larger entity, such as a family, a tribe, a clan or even gang, a culture, or a larger constellation of cultures composing societal or national identity? Frohnmayer (1992) indicates that in the United States, it is possible to identify 170 ethnic groups that all share the identity of "American."

Therapist Credentials

The literature has recognized many variables that differ across cultures with respect to the issue of the credentials of the therapist. The patient's expectations of the therapist may be influenced by beliefs about the therapist's identity on the basis of age, gender, group affiliation, and so forth. These expectations may involve the degree of intervention by the therapist, as well as the nature of treatment. Is the therapist expected to be a neutral party, friend, unquestioned authority, or co-investigator and partner in healing?

For example, West (1987) points out that in Islamic societies, "many patients believe that the therapist is *hakeem,* that is, wise man and healer, not a physician in the Western sense but a professional working through the hands of Allah" (p. 105). Thus, patients present with the expectation that the therapist will "guess their problem" and "know the answers." West (1987) further notes, "The concept to work to help the self is generally nonexistent. Their question becomes: If I can heal myself then why am I here?" (p. 106).

In contrast, Kottler et al. (1994) describe the Western therapeutic relationship as a dynamically evolving process geared toward developing a working alliance with patients on the basis of the idea of "a shared journey"; the purpose of the journey is to allow therapist and patient to diagnose and treat problems cooperatively, while avoiding dependency, which is viewed as pathological. Thus, in general, the Western view of therapist as tool or self-help aid (taken to its managed care extreme, as the "employee" of a "client") directly contradicts the Eastern view of therapist as guru. Indeed, cultures in which the concept of karma is highly valued may view the very existence of a particular therapeutic dyad as a predetermined relationship, grounded in destiny.

Age and Gender Considerations

The age and gender of the therapist may also affect the relationship. Do patients from all cultures subscribe to the "older is wiser" paradigm? Is an unmarried therapist without children seen as a failure, incapable of giving help in a culture that values marriage and procreation as integral purposes for existence? Some literature shows that in paternalistic cultures, such as Arabic or Hispanic cultures, in which males are not expected to reveal weaknesses to females, the major challenge to establishing a therapeutic relationship between a male patient and a female therapist is that disclosure of problems and seeking help from a therapist of opposite gender may jeopardize the male patient's self-esteem, which must be preserved at all costs (Comas-Diaz and Griffith 1988; Javier and Yussef 1995; Mass and Al-Krenawi 1994).

Subgroup Affiliation

In understanding cultural variables in the therapeutic relationship, the therapist's group or subgroup affiliation is a critical determinant of the patient's ability to trust the therapist. For example, among Cambodian refugees, where ethnic subgroup or political affiliation (e.g., Communist revolutionary vs. government employee) determined life or death during the genocidal regime of Pol Pot (1975–1979), the Western assumption of the therapist as patient advocate, with its implication of confidentiality, was not in accord with the Cambodian citizens' experience of authority figures having primary allegiance to the state. In this context, disclosure of information jeopardized the individual and his or her family. Gorkin (1986) describes the deleterious effects on the therapeutic relationship between Israeli therapists, who had compulsory military service and have reserve status, and Palestinian patients, who have genuine reasons rooted in life experience to distrust the Israeli military.

Concept of Illness

The therapist's credentials as healer may be influenced by the patient's model of illness (Castillo 1997; Kleinman 1980). For example, does the therapist possess the ability to harness the appropriate supernatural powers necessary for healing? Bilu and Witztum (1993) recommend that when working with ultra-orthodox Jewish patients, the therapist should be portrayed as an agent serving to execute the will of God, since God must ultimately be credited with any healing that occurs.

Patient Autonomy

The next area that must be addressed in culturally sensitive psychotherapy is the patient's identity as a patient, which includes cultural variations in the concept of autonomy. This has implications for practical issues such as therapist-patient boundaries and disclosure of confidential information. Dimou (1995) discusses the culturally valued self-image, quoting the German philosopher Max Scheler's distinction between the Western prototype of the active hero, who wants to change the world, and the Eastern prototype of the wise sage, who wants to learn the best way to endure suffering. Is the patient supposed to be active or passive, the American "Marlboro Man" taking charge of his destiny, or the Eastern Buddha-like figure enduring suffering as part of his karmic destiny? Pedder (1991) points out that the Western model would consider a patient's dependence on the therapist as pathological, a "malignant regression," while Neki (1976) reminds us that in Indian societies, dependence is a "developmental goal." Doi (1973, 1989) describes the Japanese concept of *amaeru,* defined as a culturally sanctioned relationship in adults in which one depends on the love of an other, similar to the mother-child relationship. He states that the patient-therapist relationship is defined by *amae,* which describes the patient's behaviors and affects in relating to the therapist as rooted in that of a child seeking a maternal, caring relationship. Many cultures do not assign primary importance to the individual, but rather view the individual as a representation of a larger group (Dwairy and Van Sickle 1996; Kitayama et al. 1997).

Different models of individuation have implications on disclosure in therapy. Dwairy and Van Sickle (1996) quoted an Arabic societal colloquialism, "*Alshakualgair Allah mathalla,*" meaning, "Complaining to anyone other than God is a disgrace." Similarly, many Asian societies view disclosure on the part of a patient as a betrayal of family secrets (Uba 1994). The patient is thus expected not to shame the family. Berg and Jaya (1993) point out that in Asian families, children who do not behave are threatened with banishment from the family. In the United States, children are threatened with being "grounded" and having to spend more time at home with the family! Mull (1993) cites a case among the Lao Hmong in which a therapist, who did not consult with community elders before initiating treatment, precipitated a hospital boycott by the entire Lao Hmong community. The idea that confidentiality is limited to the patient does not apply in cultures that view the family or community as more important than the individual. Blackhall et al. (1995), in their study of ethnicity and attitudes toward patient autonomy, concluded that Korean Americans and Mexican Americans were more likely to believe that the family, rather than the patient, should make medical decisions than were African American and European American subjects, who believed that the individual patient should have the necessary information to direct treatment.

Reciprocal Expectations of Therapy

Literature that focuses on the therapist's expectations of the patient, and reciprocally the patient's expectations of the therapist, has addressed the issue of culture in this dynamic. The question of what makes a "good patient" raises some general issues about Western versus Eastern biases and assumptions. For example, in working with Chinese patients, the therapist should know that Asians are expected to accept the passive role imposed by the therapist, avoid questioning or confronting an authority figure, demonstrate respect by avoiding eye contact, and not complain about treatment (Uba 1994; Wong and Piran 1995). Thus, patients are likely to avoid taking medication, rather than complaining to the psychiatrist about side effects. This "noncompliance" from the Western view is considered culturally appropriate behavior from the Eastern perspective, because it allows the patient to avoid direct confrontation with an authority figure. Wong and Piran (1995) suggest that when working with Chinese clients, "it is important to clarify that acceptance does not mean agreement" (p. 110).

Communication Styles

Carter (1995), in describing sociocultural issues in working with African Americans, cites differences in eye contact (African Americans are expected to look away while listening, which may be perceived as disinterest), facial expression, and physical touch. Some African Americans maintain a belief in the curative powers of touch ("royal touch") and may consider a therapeutic encounter incomplete without a "laying on of hands" or physical contact between the patient and healer. Thus, a physical examination is preferable to a verbal diagnostic interview. Strict Arabic cultures would view a male therapist's touching a female patient as an inappropriate sexual overture (Mass and Al-Krenawi 1994).

Therapeutic Boundaries: Disclosure, Gift-Giving, and Individuality

As noted earlier, cultural beliefs influence the patient's expectations of the therapist. Polynesian patients may expect disclosure in the form of a therapist's revealing his or her genealogy prior to establishing a trusting relationship. Chinese patients may expect the therapist to demonstrate expertise by prescribing medications; a visit to a physician that does not result in the prescription or administration of medications may not be considered effective and may call into question the knowledge or skills of the therapist.

The issue of whether a patient is expected to give a gift to the therapist, and whether or not the therapist is expected to accept the gift, is replete with potential for culture-based misinterpretation. In countries such as Japan, where gift giving is considered an art, and where the wrapping may convey more value than the gift itself (Berg and Jaya 1993), refusing a gift may be seen as a harsh rejection of the patient or family on the part of the therapist. In Polynesian cultures, the patient may expect the sharing of food or drink during the clinical encounter. Failure to participate in this experience with the patient may be viewed as a therapeutic rejection that can severely damage rapport.

The purpose or outcome of therapy must also reflect cultural expectations. For example, Kitayama et al. (1997, p. 1246) point out that while "numerous studies conducted in North America in recent decades have demonstrated a robust and pervasive tendency to maintain and enhance an overall evaluation of the self—self esteem," this therapeutic goal is not necessarily generalizable to Asians: "In sharp contrast, however, there is a growing body of studies that indicate that such a self-enhancing effect is greatly attenuated and, in some cases, completely reversed in non-Western, especially Asian, groups." Dwairy and Van Sickle (1996) point out that because Arabic societies discourage individualism and prefer maintenance of the rigid familial hierarchy, "the Arabic patient who has experienced a 'successful' course of treatment in Western psychotherapy will also experience its iatrogenic effects; specifically, greater familial and social conflict. In such cases the alleviation of the internal conflict will result in a new external conflict" (p. 236).

Defining Illness and Treatment

The culturally sensitive therapist must realize that the patient's culture imposes expectations on the therapist. For example, in Chinese culture, the therapist is expected to make the diagnosis and does not necessarily need input from the patient. The therapist should know the appropriate treatment and impose it, not negotiate it with the patient, a process that may be seen as a sign of weakness or therapeutic incompetence (Kottler et al. 1994). The patient may arrive with a diagnosis that has been predetermined by the community, such as one of the culture-bound syndromes like *dhat* (or semen loss) among Indians or *hwa-byung* (fire sickness), an anger syndrome that includes somatic complaints, among the Koreans. In such cases, the therapist who questions the diagnosis runs the risk of offending the community in which the patient functions. As noted earlier, the therapist who does not disclose information to Lao Hmong community elders, or who enters into a treatment relationship with a Lao Hmong patient without the approval of community elders, can risk community ostracism.

Ethnic and Cultural Transference

A large body of literature has been devoted to the study of the applicability of the psychodynamic framework to patients of varying cultures. The concept of transference brings with it certain nosological conundrums. Concepts such as therapeutic resistance, the presence or absence of unconscious defense mechanisms particular to certain cultures, and even the presence of an "ethnic unconscious" (Herron 1995) are important in understanding the nature of the therapeutic relationship from a cultural perspective. How does one distinguish countertransference from prejudice related to the patient's religion, ethnicity, nationality, or even body habitus (Ingram 1978)?

The cultural aspects of transference and countertransference have been addressed mainly in the psychoanalytic literature. A variety of psychoanalytic literature is dedicated to exploring whether the psychoanalytic model is applicable across cultures, or how it must be modified when used with patients from specific cultures (Kakar 1985; Ng 1985; Spiegel 1988). As Comaz-Diaz and Jacobsen (1991) point out, ethnocultural transference and countertransference occur within the context of a "therapeutic dyad" consisting of the therapist and the patient. This dyadic relationship can be examined from a variety of perspectives, including a focus on problems that occur when there is similarity or dissonance between the ethnocultural backgrounds of the patient and therapist.

Transference and Countertransference: Definitions

Before examining these issues, one must start with definitions of transference and countertransference, which are themselves problematic. In the narrow psychoanalytic definition, Freud described *countertransference* as "the unconscious counterreaction to the patient's transference, indicative of the therapist's own unresolved intrapsychic conflicts" (Slakter 1987, p. 88). Freud cautioned that "no psychoanalyst goes further than his own complexes and internal resistances permit" (Slakter 1987, p. 88). *Transference* was described by Freud as the unconscious reaction a patient has toward a therapist, which was believed to be rooted in antecedents from childhood. Subsequent psychoanalytic literature identified multiple subtypes of transference, such as positive, negative, erotic, and psychotic, with countertransference implications for each.

The broad view of transference and countertransference—the view that will be addressed in this chapter—refers to transference as encompassing all feelings patients have toward therapists, and countertransference as encompassing all feelings therapists have toward patients. It is useful to analyze some fundamental concepts of the psychoanalytic view in attempting to discuss the cultural variables inherent in the therapeutic relationship.

Psychodynamics and Relationship Boundaries

As noted earlier, although psychoanalysis treats the patient-therapist relationship as dyadic, it is really a relationship that exists on many levels. At one level is the nature of the patient's relationship with the larger framework of culture, which extends beyond the patient as an individual and may include others (e.g., parents, tribal elders). Psychodynamic theory places primacy on the idea of therapeutic neutrality. When working with patients of paternalistic cultures, such as the Islamic culture of the Bedouin (Mass and Al-Krenawi 1994) or traditional Arabic societies (Dwairy and Van Sickle 1996), the therapist is advised to be active in creating a pseudofamilial relationship with the patient. This nature of this relationship varies depending on the patient's age, sex, and social status. This approach preserves the hierarchical relationship of the family. Dwairy and Van Sickle (1996, p. 244) state that "in essence, authority figures of the family are treated as partners whose cooperation and support is essential for the success of the treatment," and they caution that "the message to the family must be: 'Nothing can be changed without your permission and assistance.'" In a pseudofamilial relationship, in which the therapist is seen as a wise relative, the problems posed when patient and therapist are of different gender are obviated, since sexual relationships would never be expected to occur within this structure.

Problems Arising From Application of Psychodynamic Theory Across Cultures

Kakar (1985) points out that dynamic constructs, such as libidinal drives that culminate in an oedipal crisis, may not be applicable to Indian culture. Kakar further notes that the very notion of an unconscious root of conflict that manifests as pathology is not applicable in cultures, such as those of India, in which fatalism, or paying off of karmic debt, is seen as a causative agent of problems in life. In contrast to the Western psychoanalytic model, "individuality is not given at birth but is an achievement of the final stage of the life cycle when the person ideally becomes a 'renouncer' and succeeds in detaching himself from his human ties and relationships" (Kakar 1985, p. 445).

Some theorists posit an "ethnic unconscious," which "refers to material that is derived from identification with a particular group of people who have sufficient characteristics in common to give themselves a categorical name" (Herron 1995, p. 525). The implication is that every culture has defensive hierarchies that result in cultural patterns, and a "commonality of defenses" that give rise to a particular ethnic character. Taken to a somewhat less theoretical level, the therapist is challenged with knowing when reactions toward a particular patient are rooted in common stereotypes and prejudices rather than complex intrapsychic conflicts that produce countertransference reactions.

Variations of Ethnocultural Transference and Countertransference

Perhaps the best analysis of cultural issues identified with transference and countertransference in therapy currently available is that of Comas-Diaz and Jacobsen (1991). They dissect the therapeutic dyad into the categories of *inter*ethnic transference (patient and therapist are of different backgrounds), *intra*ethnic transference (patient and therapist are from the same ethnic background), and their interethnic and intraethnic complementary countertransference reactions. Transference can occur in many variations, including overcompliance, excessive admiration, denial of the importance of ethnicity, suspicion of therapist motives, stereotype projections based on ethnicity, and hostility. Countertransference reactions can include inappropriate exploration based on curiosity, guilt grounded in perceived collusion with the oppressive majority, denial of the therapeutic importance of ethnocultural differences ("cultural myopia"), and aggression based on prejudice. Countertransference reactions rooted in an intraethnic therapeutic relationship can include feelings of survivor guilt, overidentification, and defensive distancing.

Although the analysis by Comas-Diaz and Jacobsen (1991) is useful, it is not exhaustive. Other mental health practitioners and theorists have identified additional types of transference and countertransference reactions influenced by culture. For example, in a candid discussion of his own psychoanalysis, Taketomo (1989) describes a phenomenon called "teacher transference." His formative education in the Japanese school system fostered a paternal transference response toward his training analyst, which he believes was rooted in the Japanese view of the teacher as parental authority.

In their analysis of intracultural countertransference, Comas-Diaz and Jacobsen (1991) underemphasized the real differences in subcultures within the same society. Such differences may take the form of discrimination against a minority caste on the basis of its historical occupation or livelihood within the dominant culture. For example, a Japanese therapist working with a Japanese patient who is *Burakumin* (a minority subgroup of Japanese deemed "untouchable" because of their historical role in Japanese society as leather workers, who are therefore *eta,* or "contaminated," because of their contact with dead animals) may have culturally sanctioned feelings of prejudice.

In present-day Japan, families commonly do an extensive genealogical investigation of potential marriage partners to ensure that a family member is not marrying a member of the *Burakumin* caste, since no physical characteristics distinguish *Burakumin* from majority Japanese. The influence of Buddhism, with its prohibitions against contact with corpses, likely influenced the historical evolution of this so-called lower caste. A similar discrimination between subgroups within the same ethnic group exists between the majority Han Chinese in Taiwan and Guandong, China, and the *Hakka* minority (also known as *Ke Ren,* or guest people). The *Hakka* were stigmatized by their historical migration south as war refugees from central China, gaining the name of guest people from the *bendi* (local people), as the original population called itself.

Suggestions for Therapists

As indicated earlier, the therapeutic relationship is replete with opportunities for misunderstanding that can compromise the efficacy of treatment. The following are suggestions for the therapist who may encounter some of the challenges of culturally sensitive treatment.

1. *Become familiar with the culture, subculture, and political history of the patient when these differ from those of the therapist.* Although it would be impossible for a therapist to gain the degree of cultural insight that an anthropologist or historian may have, investing some time to develop a basic grasp of these issues yields valuable rewards. First, it gives the therapist a contextual understanding of the patient that will be useful in avoiding the common therapeutic blunder of overgeneralization. For example, when working with patients from Vietnam, knowing their ethnicity (some Vietnamese are ethnically Chinese), political affiliation in their country of origin (oppressed minority vs. empowered majority), religious beliefs (some Vietnamese are Christians who lived in a majority Buddhist country), and expectations of gender roles all contribute to providing the therapist a more precise framework from which therapy can be applied. In other words, the therapist will appreciate that being Vietnamese is not an all-encompassing cultural descriptor for patients from Vietnam. A second benefit is that patients usually will recognize and appreciate the therapist's attempt to learn about their culture, and this enhances the therapeutic alliance.

2. *Recognize that because the concept of boundaries varies across cultures, therapeutic elements related to boundaries must be modified to adapt to this variance.* For example, do not assume that confidentiality is implicitly restricted to the therapist and the designated patient. In many cultures, confidentiality is neither expected nor therapeutic.

3. *Recognize that the patient is part of a larger cultural context.* Representatives of this larger system, which may include family members, societal elders, and so forth, may be enlisted as therapeutic allies, or they may be alienated, with disastrous results to the therapy. For example, when working with Arabic families, which operate along a well-defined hierarchical structure, the therapist is advised to create a pseudofamilial relationship in which he or she is a member, rather than attempting therapy on the basis of the concept of a two-person (dyadic) relationship. The strictly dyadic relationship may cause the patient to become alienated from his or her cultural supports.

4. *Recognize that common issues in the therapeutic relationship, such as gifts, touch, eye contact, medication compliance, and choice of vocabulary, are all influenced by culture.* The therapist is advised not to adhere to any rigid theoretical approach to dealing with these phenomena; rather, the therapist is advised to seek out the cultural meaning of these issues on a case-specific basis. When necessary, the therapist should enlist the expertise of a "cultural informant." This person is generally from the

same culture as the patient, is not an active participant in the therapy, and functions as a consultant to the therapist by interpreting or identifying culture-specific issues. In this manner, the efficacy of the therapist is enhanced.

5. *Recognize that the therapeutic paradigm (e.g., psychodynamic) must be flexible.* The degree of active intervention by the therapist, definition of therapeutic goals, techniques used, and outcome measures must all be modified to reflect cultural differences in the therapy.

6. *Recognize that transference and countertransference interactions influenced by culture will occur.* Be familiar with the common varieties of interethnic and intraethnic transference and countertransference reactions that occur in therapy. Recognize that phenomena such as cultural stereotyping often occur even when the therapist and patient share the same ethnocultural background.

The psychotherapeutic relationship is complex and operates on many overlapping levels. The therapist and the patient bring to the relationship a panoply of sociocultural beliefs and behaviors. Together they share the challenge of forming a therapeutic alliance, identifying a problem, and working toward a solution that may have implications beyond the traditionally defined therapeutic dyad. The therapist who works from a culturally sensitive framework must be prepared to identify problems and modify his or her therapeutic repertoire to meet the challenges imposed by this meeting of minds and cultures.

References

Berg KI, Jaya A: Different and same: family therapy with Asian-American families. J Marital Fam Ther 19:31–38, 1993

Bilu Y, Witztum E: Working with Jewish ultra-orthodox patients: guidelines for a culturally sensitive therapy. Cult Med Psychiatry 17:197–235, 1993

Blackhall LJ, Murphy ST, Frank G, et al: Ethnicity and attitudes toward patient autonomy. JAMA 274:820–825, 1995

Carter J: Psychosocial/cultural issues in medicine and psychiatry: treating African Americans. J Natl Med Assoc 87:857–860, 1995

Castillo RJ: Culture and Mental Illness: A Client-Centered Approach. Pacific Grove, CA, Brooks/Cole, 1997

Comas-Diaz L, Griffith EEH: Clinical Guidelines in Cross-Cultural Mental Health. New York, Wiley, 1988

Comas-Diaz L, Jacobsen F: Ethnocultural transference and countertransference in the therapeutic dyad. Am J Orthopsychiatry 61:392–402, 1991

Dimou N: Illness and culture: learning differences. Patient Education and Counseling 26:153–157, 1995

Doi T: The Anatomy of Dependence: The Key Analysis of Japanese Behavior. Tokyo, Kodansha International, 1973

Doi T: The concept of amae and its psychoanalytic implications. International Review of Psychoanalysis 16:349–354, 1989

Dwairy M, Van Sickle T: Western psychotherapy in traditional Arabic societies. Clin Psychol Rev 16:231–249, 1996

Frohnmayer JE: Is that what he meant? New York Times, June 14, 1992, E19

Gorkin M: Countertransference in cross-cultural psychotherapy: the example of Jewish therapist and Arab patient. Psychiatry 49:69–79, 1986

Herron W: Development of the ethnic unconscious. Psychoanalytic Psychology 12:521–532, 1995

Ingram D: Cultural counterresistance in the analytic treatment of the obese woman. Am J Psychoanal 38:155–161, 1978

Javier R, Yussef M: A Latino perspective on the role of ethnicity in the development of moral values: implications for psychoanalytic theory and practice. J Am Acad Psychoanal 23:79–97, 1995

Kakar S: Psychoanalysis and non-western cultures. International Review of Psycho-analysis 12:441–448, 1985

Kitayama S, Markus HR, Matsumoto H, et al: Individual and collective process in the construction of the self: self-enhancement in the United States and self-criticism in Japan. J Pers Soc Psychol 72:1245–1267, 1997

Kleinman A: Patients and Healers in the Context of Culture: An Exploration of the Borderland Between Anthropology, Medicine, and Psychiatry. Berkeley, University of California Press, 1980

Kottler J, Sexton T, Whiston S: The Heart of Healing: Relationships in Therapy. San Francisco, CA, Jossey-Bass, 1994

Mass M, Al-Krenawi A: When a man encounters a woman, Satan is also present: clinical relationships. Am J Orthopsychiatry 64:357–367, 1994

Mull DJ: Cross-cultural communication in the physician's office. West J Med 159:609–613, 1993

Neki JS: An examination of the cultural relativism of dependence as a dynamic of social and therapeutic relationships. Br J Med Psychol 49:1–22, 1976

Ng ML: Psychoanalysis for the Chinese: applicable or not applicable? International Review of Psychoanalysis 12:449–460, 1985

Pedder J: Fear of dependence in therapeutic relationships. Br J Med Psychol 64:117–126, 1991

Ridley C: Pseudo-transference in interracial psychotherapy: an operant paradigm. Journal of Contemporary Psychotherapy 15:29–36, 1985

Slakter E: Countertransference. Northvale, NJ, Jason Aronson, 1987

Spiegel J: The effect of strangeness in psychoanalysis. Contemporary Psychoanalysis 24:379–391, 1988

Taketomo Y: An American-Japanese transcultural psychoanalysis and the issue of teacher transference. J Am Acad Psychoanal 17:427–450, 1989

Uba L: Asian Americans: Personality Patterns, Identity, and Mental Health. New York, Guilford, 1994

West J: Psychotherapy in the eastern province of Saudi Arabia. Psychotherapy 24:105–107, 1987

Wong OC, Piran N: Western biases and assumptions as impediments in counseling traditional Chinese clients. Canadian Journal of Counseling 29:107–119, 1995

Yi K: Psychoanalytic psychotherapy with Asian clients: transference and therapeutic considerations. Psychotherapy 32:309–317, 1995

CHAPTER 9

Psychological Aspects of Giving and Receiving Medications

Iqbal Ahmed, M.D.

Dramatic developments in psychopharmacology over the past several decades have led to the frequent practice of combining psychotherapy with the prescription of medications. In addition to the biological effects of medicines, the prescription process has psychological implications that influence the doctor-patient relationship and other aspects of the psychotherapy. Culture can be a powerful determinant of these psychological implications. Additionally, cultural factors influence the belief in, and response to, medications. Thus, in this chapter, cultural dimensions of medication prescription are elaborated in relation to the process of psychotherapy.

Clinical experience reveals that various racial/ethnic groups respond differently to medication treatments. Biological, psychological, and sociocultural factors that account for this variation in response include different pharmacokinetics among the groups that are determined by genetics or other biological factors; different dietary practices observed among different ethnic groups; different patterns of patients' illness behavior, including different culturally determined attitudes toward medication consumption; and variations in physicians' prescribing practices (Turner and Cooley-Quille 1996).

Ethnicity and Biological Response

Race and ethnicity affect the pharmacodynamics and pharmacokinetics of medications, including psychotropic agents (Lin et al. 1995). Drug interactions that are mediated by the cytochrome P450 system vary among racial/ ethnic groups because of genetic differences. Several studies reported in the psychiatric literature have examined the effect of ethnicity, but there has been a paucity of information on the effect of culture on the clinical response of patients to prescribed medications. Culture and symbolic processes may have potent effects on psychiatric treatment outcome (Kleinman 1988). In fact, these processes may determine, to a large extent, the clinical effects of psychotropics, as well as other medications, rather than their real pharmacological properties.

   Direct biological effects of culturally determined behavior, such as diet, may also affect a patient's response to medication. A few studies have demonstrated that diet affects cross-ethnic differences in drug metabolism (Lin et al. 1995). When Asian-Indian immigrants switched from a traditional vegetarian diet to a British diet, their drug pharmacokinetics became similar to those of Caucasian-British subjects (Allen et al. 1977; Fraser et al. 1979).

Nonbiological Influences of
Culture on Medication Response

Culture has nonbiological effects on medication response that are due to factors such as patient compliance, placebo effects of medications, and other behaviors affecting drug interactions (interaction of dietary habits and alternative treatments such as herbal remedies). Since noncompliance is reported in over 50% of patients, and the placebo response can account for about 30% of a drug's effects, the role of culture on these effects becomes a significant but understudied phenomenon. The intervening variables in these nonbiological effects are related to the patient, the doctor, and their relationship

(Smith et al. 1993); cultural beliefs about illness and medication; and the actual process of giving and receiving medications. The influence of culture on each of these variables is examined in brief here.

The Patient

Culture may affect the patient in various ways, such as through personality and behavior patterns; perception of stress and coping style, including manner of utilization of social support; and interaction, including transference, with the doctor. These variables will influence the process and outcome of medical treatment, including medication response.

The patient's personality development is affected by culture, which in turn may influence the reaction toward medication (Lin et al. 1995). On the basis of an international survey of clinicians, Murphy (1969) suggested that patients from cultures that give strong emphasis to independence, struggle, and action (typically Euro-American culture) are likely to require more medication than patients whose personalities are shaped by cultures that emphasize interdependence and social adaptation (typically Asian cultures). Subsequent research suggested that, even among Asian cultures, persons from ethnic groups that are more action-oriented and aggressive, such as Chinese (compared with Malays, for example), are more resistant to neuroleptics in the treatment of schizophrenia. Among Euro-American cultures, the less aggressive and action-oriented French Canadians were more vulnerable to side effects of anxiolytics than were Anglo-Canadians (Murphy 1972).

Reactions to stress and utilization of social support are thought to be important factors affecting medication response (needing different dosages and levels of medications) and prognosis of illness. For example, higher levels of "expressed emotion" (frequent criticism, hostility, and emotional over-involvement) in families of patients with schizophrenia are associated with poorer response to medications (Falloon and Liberman 1983; Vaughn and Leff 1976). There appear to be different levels of expressed emotions in different cultural groups (Lin et al. 1995). Anglo-American families have been reported to have higher levels of expressed emotions than British families, who, in turn, have higher levels of expressed emotions than Hispanic families.

Patient role is prescribed by culture, especially in relating to the physician and complying with treatment recommendations. There might be unique transference toward the physician related to the perceived cultural orientation of the doctor (e.g., traditional healer or Western trained), based on racial and power relationships. Patient role and transference, in turn, affect the beliefs and expectations about the relationship with, and treatments prescribed by, the physician.

The Doctor

Culture influences the doctor's prescribing habits and decisions in several ways, including the doctor's role and "healing power," desire to please the patient (e.g., providing a placebo), countertransference (including biases about race and ethnicity), and professional norms and values (Higginbotham and Streiner 1991; van der Geest and Whyte 1988). Physicians work within the context of competing demands from patients, colleagues, governmental agencies, and pharmaceutical companies. Even when doctors do not see a medical need to prescribe medicines, they may do so to comply with patient demands, and thus placate the patient.

Doctors may also be affected by their perceptions of a patient's illness, based on racial or ethnic characteristics. This can influence their diagnosis of the illness and beliefs about likely treatment response. They might perceive patients from certain ethnic backgrounds as having more psychopathology, as being more likely to need medications (rather than psychotherapy), as needing more "potent" medications (with more adverse effects), and as having a worse prognosis for their illness. Doctors have been found to over-pathologize symptoms found in African Americans and Hispanics, and possibly to minimize symptoms in Caucasians (Lopez 1989). For example, among Caucasian psychiatrists, African American patients were more likely to be diagnosed as having schizophrenia and to be treated with antipsychotic drugs than were Caucasian patients, who were diagnosed with mood disorders, even when both had similar symptoms (Simon et al. 1973; Turner and Cooley-Quille 1996).

The Illness

Culture influences etiological conceptions and the symbolic meaning of illness. Etiological concepts include natural/supernatural, reductionistic/holistic, and biological/nonbiological distinctions. Illness is also interpreted in psychological or spiritual terms, in terms of humoral theory (bile, blood, phlegm) or hot-cold theory of disease, as patterns of energy flow (such as *chi*), and as problems of balance of forces (such as *yin* and *yang*). The greater the disparity between contemporary scientific concepts of disease and the patient's traditional folk beliefs about illness, the greater the likelihood of noncompliance.

Believing in *yin-yang* balance of the universe and the need for the same in the body, some Asian patients, and more recently Westerners, may combine herbs with Western psychotropic drugs without telling their psychiatrists (Chien 1993). In general, more and more people are using herbal remedies and other alternative treatments along with Western medications, both in the United States and elsewhere in the world. This can be seen in the widespread use of agents such as Saint-John's-wort, ginseng, gingko biloba, and kava kava. Asians (and even many Westerners) hold the belief that Eastern herbal drugs are not as harmful or toxic as Western modern medicines. However, these agents are pharmacologically active, have both therapeutic and toxic effects, and can lead to both pharmacokinetic and pharmacodynamic drug-drug interactions with Western medications (Crone and Wise 1998).

Beliefs (such as the hot-cold theory of disease) about drug-disease interactions (e.g., needing a cold drug for a hot disease and a hot drug for a cold disease) can affect compliance and perceived efficacy of medications. Puerto Rican patients may stop taking prophylactic penicillin, thought to be a hot drug, for rheumatic fever if they have concomitant diarrhea, which is considered a hot disease (Harwood 1971). In Jamaica, hypertension is viewed by laypersons as being caused by worrying and improper circulation of blood. Consequently, the desirable medication is one that cools the blood and the person as a whole. Antihypertensive medications are not viewed as being "effective" because they do not produce the proper sensation (Higginbotham and Streiner 1991). On the other hand, people in many societies, including the United States, seem to believe that medication need not be used or should be stopped as soon as symptoms disappear. This is commonly seen in the form of noncompliance with antihypertensive medications.

The Meaning of Medication

Cultures may objectify healing through medicines. Medicines facilitate particular social and symbolic processes (van der Geest and Whyte 1988, 1989). This may be considered the "symbolic" effect of medication, compared with the pharmacological or "instrumental" effect. The symbolic effect includes imbued characteristics, such as the "life" or "healing power" of a drug, and the attribution of value. Patients may experience and associate certain emotions with the use of certain medications. Medication can be viewed as a metaphor (e.g., for more personal autonomy). Studies reporting how these symbolic effects might be based on cultural beliefs about characteristics of the medications and about alternative treatments have been reviewed by other authors (Higginbotham and Streiner 1991; van der Geest and Whyte 1988, 1989). These beliefs, in turn, have an impact on both compliance and placebo response. The following are some of the characteristics of medicines that may have cultural meaning.

Form or Consistency

Form or consistency refers to the physical characteristics (e.g., tablet, capsule, or liquid), color, size, amount, and even the name of the medicine. These characteristics may all have different implications regarding the potency or power of the medication in a particular culture. The color of capsules has been reported to affect placebo response differentially in different ethnic groups. For instance, white capsules were viewed by Caucasians as analgesics and by African Americans as stimulants. On the other hand, black capsules were viewed by Caucasians as stimulants and by African Americans as analgesics (Buckalew and Coffield 1982). Yellow pills are seen as suitable against depression in Europe, and red capsules are appropriate modes of strengthening the blood in Sierra Leone (van der Geest and Whyte 1988). Similarly, within the context of the hot-cold theory of disease and the Ayurvedic system of medicine, colors and forms of medicine may have quite different indications and meanings for the patient than for the physician (Nichter 1980). Culture may also affect the amount of medication bought by patients. In El Salvador, patients buy pills in multiples of four, since the number has ritual significance.

Sensation Experienced

The sensation experienced refers to the reaction that occurs after the medication is taken, including the taste, such as bitter or sweet. Bitter medications are believed in some cultures to be more potent and effective. Certain types of aftertastes are considered indicative of the effect of the medication, either therapeutic or averse, in some folk systems of medicine (Nichter 1980).

Source of Medicine

Whether the medicine is derived from plants, is derived from animals, or is synthetic can have a psychological impact on medication response. For instance, because of religious proscriptions, Moslems may not use alcohol-containing liquid medications, and they and orthodox Jews may not use medications containing porcine products. Vegetarians may not be willing to take medications with animal products in them. Patients might not always share reasons for noncompliance with physicians with different beliefs.

Other issues related to sources of medication include whether the manufacture is domestic or foreign, and the degree of difficulty in obtaining the medicine. Western medicines may be viewed as potent, faster, and superior for acute illness, whereas herbal medicines are seen as milder, slower, and better for chronic illness. The Indochinese believe that medication should be taken only during the acute phase of illness, and for a short time. Chronic use is feared as leading to dependence and being harmful to the body (Kroll et al. 1990). In India, "English" medications may be viewed as being more potent than traditional Ayurvedic ones and, therefore, may be used only to a limited extent with the very young and the very old, who are too weak to tolerate these agents.

Packaging

The presentation of the medicine—whether it is modern and scientific-looking, and whether the site of manufacture and distribution is the physician's office, a dispensary, or a pharmacy—can influence the patient's perception of its value and perceived efficacy. The traditional belief in Eastern herbal medicines, which consist of several herbs, has accustomed Asians to polypharmacy. Physicians in Japan, Korea, China, and Taiwan often use polypharmacy as standard practice, and they usually do not disclose the contents of medicines to patients (Chien 1993). The philosophy behind this practice is that mystery of the contents gives more therapeutic power to the treatment. Several medications of different colors and forms may be given in a single package. Such polypharmacy is widely accepted by patients, who believe a good doctor is skillful in combining different kinds of drugs.

Mode of Administration

Injectable agents are often thought to be more potent than oral. Popularity of injections is particularly noticeable in developing countries (Reeler 1990). A number of reasons for this have been speculated. Visible crossing of the body limits with the needle, combined with the ritual of filling the syringe, may be perceived as invoking the help of powerful outside healing forces. In addition, the experience of pain from the injection may be perceived as a sign of the potency of the treatment.

Giving and Receiving Medication

The critical exchange (the transaction) of prescribing medication and receiving it involves a great deal of psychology. Cultural beliefs, attitudes, and values of both the patient and the physician affect the exchange. Culture influences the nature of the doctor-patient relationship and the symbolic meaning of the transaction itself for all parties involved (patient, doctor, family, and so on). To this transaction, patients bring culturally shaped expectations about desirable medications for their illness experience, and the doctor brings a mixture of clinical, cultural, and commercial motives (Higginbotham and Streiner 1991).

The transaction between doctor and patient has both material and symbolic aspects. Material aspects of the transaction include the prescription or the transfer of medications with their inherent pharmacological properties, including both the pharmacological therapeutic and adverse effects, as well as the monetary value of the transaction. The symbolic meaning of the transaction for the doctor might include demonstrating culturally sanctioned power, such as the symbolic transfer of love, or spiritual potency (e.g., from shamans). To maintain his or her power, the doctor may keep the ingredients secret or may not explain their pharmacological effects. In current Western practice, the doctor describes the ingredients and discloses their therapeutic and adverse effects (informed consent).

For the patient, the symbolic meaning of the transaction might include being fed, cared for, accepted, and even loved. Whereas in some Western countries, such as the United States, taking medications may be viewed as a loss of autonomy and a sign of weakness, in other countries and cultures it may be perceived quite differently. Medications may be viewed as substances with innate powers that may be acquired by an individual. This enables therapy to be "liberated" from social relationships, in which it would otherwise be embedded (van der Geest and Whyte 1988). By receiving powerful medicine, the patient may believe that strength to combat powerful illness is being transferred from the doctor. The ensuing negotiations in this context determine the prescription practices of the physician, the compliance with the prescription, and the patient's experience of the pharmacological and placebo effects of the medication.

Noncompliance may be more common among non-Western populations in the United States (Smith et al. 1993). This increased noncompliance may be due to different beliefs about illness and treatment. The risk of noncompliance is compounded when there are communication difficulties about these differences. Medication compliance might be a particularly serious problem in cross-cultural settings (Kinzie et al. 1987). Socioeconomic factors such as education, cost, and access to care may also contribute to noncompliance. Another factor may be different prescribing habits by providers. African Americans with psychosis were prescribed higher doses of antipsychotic medications and more "as needed" (prn) medications, resulting in more adverse effects, poorer patient compliance, and delays in seeking treatment (Lawson 1996; Sellwood and Tarrier 1994). All these factors may contribute to why African American and other minorities may have poorer outcomes and are more often placed on injectable depot antipsychotic medications.

Medication Usage and Efficacy

Culture influences medication usage and efficacy through the placebo effect, compliance, and drug interactions (with diet and herbal remedies). The symbolic meaning of the medication to the patient affects the placebo response and treatment compliance. There is some evidence that placebo response may be more prominent in non-Caucasians (Escobar and Tuason 1980; Goldberg et al. 1966). Culturally determined beliefs and expectations also appear to affect the perception, interpretation, and reporting of side effects. In one study of Hong Kong Chinese patients on lithium, only a very small percentage reported the typically bothersome side effects of polydipsia and polyuria to be annoying (Lee 1993). Most of them experienced these effects as positive, because they believed that water consumption and excretion are conducive to ridding the body of toxins and aiding digestion.

Culture also affects the appraisal of efficacy. Giving or prescribing of medication by physicians is based on their appraisal of "proven clinical efficacy," and the usage of medication by patients is based on the "perceived efficacy" of the medication (Higginbotham and Streiner 1991). Patients perceive efficacy according to both instrumental, or pharmacological, effects and symbolic effects of the medications. In contrast, a Western-trained doctor may look only at the proven clinical efficacy of the particular medication for the diagnosed disease. Patients evaluate the effectiveness of the medication not in terms of disease, but in terms of illness, such as the ability to cope more effectively with family, job, and neighbors. Perceived efficacy may be influenced by a number of factors, such as the illness model for the patient, perception of the power of the medication (based on its physical characteristics), perception of the healing power of the physician, or the nature of the doctor-patient relationship.

Recommendations

In view of the pervasive influence of culture on the giving and receiving of all medications, including psychopharmacological agents, the following recommendations are made with regard to the psychotherapeutic aspects of prescribing medication.

1. Take into account the following issues in determining the prescription in order to enhance compliance:

    a. The patient's concept of the illness, as well as the symbolic meaning of the illness in the patient's culture
    b. Medication characteristics, which may be important to the patient
    c. The symbolic power and value of the medication in the patient's culture
    d. Dietary habits and alternative treatments used by the patient and their potential for interactions
    e. The doctor-patient relationship, including expectations and symbolic meaning of giving and receiving medication, as well as other "transferential" aspects of the relationship

2. Negotiate with the patient, if necessary, on these issues.
3. Examine your role, values, expectations, and countertransference from your own cultural perspective, as well as the patient's.

References

Allen JJ, Rack PH, Vaddadi KS: Differences in the effects of clomipramine on English and Asian volunteers: preliminary report on a pilot study. Postgrad Med J 53 (suppl 4):79–86, 1977

Buckalew LW, Coffield KE: Drug expectations associated with perceptual characteristics: ethnic factors. Percept Mot Skills 55:915–918, 1982

Chien CP: Ethnopsychopharmacology, in Culture, Ethnicity, and Mental Illness. Edited by Gaw AC. Washington, DC, American Psychiatric Press, 1993, pp 413–430

Crone CC, Wise TN: Use of herbal medicines among consultation-liaison populations. Psychosomatics 39:3–13, 1998

Escobar JI, Tuason VB: Antidepressant agents: a cross cultural study. Psychopharmacol Bull 16:49–52, 1980

Falloon IRH, Liberman RP: Interactions between drug and psychosocial therapy in schizophrenia. Schizophr Bull 9:343–354, 1983

Fraser HS, Mucklow JC, Bulpitt CJ, et al: Environmental factors affecting antipyrine metabolism in London factory workers. Br J Clin Pharmacol 7:237–243, 1979

Goldberg SC, Schooler NR, Davidson EM, et al: Sex and race differences in response to drug treatment among schizophrenics. Psychopharmacologia 9:31–47, 1966

Harwood A: The hot-cold theory of disease: implications for treatment of Puerto Rican patients. JAMA 216:1153–1158, 1971

Higginbotham N, Streiner DL: The social science contributions to pharmacoepidemiology. J Clin Epidemiol 44 (suppl):73S–82S, 1991

Kinzie JD, Leung P, Boehnlein J, et al: Tricyclic antidepressant plasma levels in Indochinese refugees: clinical implications. J Nerv Ment Dis 175:480–485, 1987

Kleinman A: Rethinking Psychiatry. New York, Free Press, 1988

Kroll J, Linde P, Habenicht M, et al: Medication compliance, antidepressant blood levels and side effects in Southeast Asian patients. J Clin Psychopharmacol 10: 279–282, 1990

Lawson WB: Clinical issues in the pharmacotherapy of African Americans. Psychopharmacol Bull 32:275–281, 1996

Lee S: Side effects of chronic lithium therapy in Hong Kong Chinese: an ethnopsychiatric perspective. Cult Med Psychiatry 17:301–320, 1993

Lin KM, Poland RE, Anderson D: Psychopharmacology, ethnicity and culture. Transcultural Psychiatric Research Review 28:3–37, 1995

Lopez SR: Patient variable biases in clinical judgment: conceptual overview and methodological considerations. Psychol Bull 106:184–203, 1989

Murphy HBM: Ethnic variations in drug responses. Transcultural Psychiatric Research Review 6:6–23, 1969

Murphy HBM: Psychopharmacologie et variations ethnoculturelles. Confrontation Psychiatrique 9:163–185, 1972

Nichter M: The layperson's perception of medicine as perspective into the utilization of multiple therapy systems in the Indian context. Soc Sci Med 14B:225–233, 1980

Reeler AV: Injections: a fatal attraction. Soc Sci Med 31:1119–1125, 1990

Sellwood W, Tarrier N: Demographic factors associated with extreme non-compliance in schizophrenia. Soc Psychiatry Psychiatr Epidemiol 29:172–177, 1994

Simon RJ, Fleis JL, Gurland BJ, et al: Depression and schizophrenia in black and white mental patients. Arch Gen Psychiatry 28:509–512, 1973

Smith M, Lin KM, Mendoza R: "Non-biological" issues affecting psychopharmacotherapy, in Cultural Considerations, Psychopharmacology, and Psychobiology of Ethnicity. Edited by Lin KM, Poland RE, Nagasaki G. Washington, DC, American Psychiatric Press, 1993, pp 37–58

Turner SM, Cooley-Quille MR: Socioecological and sociocultural variables in psychopharmacological research: methodological considerations. Psychopharmacol Bull 30:183–192, 1996

van der Geest S, Whyte SR (eds): The Context of Medicines in Developing Countries: Studies in Pharmaceutical Anthropology. Boston, MA, Kluwer Academic, 1988

van der Geest S, Whyte SR: The charm of medicines: metaphors and metonyms. Med Anthropol Q 3:345–367, 1989

Vaughn CE, Leff JP: The influence of family and social factors on the course of psychiatric illness: a comparison of schizophrenic and depressed neurotic patients. Br J Psychiatry 129:123–137, 1976

PART 4

Treating
Special Populations

CHAPTER 10

The African American

Howard C. Blue, M.D.
Ezra E.H. Griffith, M.D.

Introduction: African American Identity

Who or what is an African American? It is a question that seems simplistic and the answer to which seems almost reflexively obvious. Yet, what constitutes African American identity is exceedingly complex. Is it race or ethnicity? Is it a matter of self-definition, or is there a purely biological basis for it? Is it a matter of sociology, politics, culture, or psychology? Indeed, it is all of these and more.

Most social scientists have rejected the notion of race as a purely biological variable (Carter 1995). Race is best understood as a sociopolitical construct, the meaning of which is derived from prevailing societal attitudes that are invested in defining and characterizing differences between people. *Ethnicity*, a term frequently interchanged with race, refers to aggregate groups of people who share common factors, such as cultural traditions, history, beliefs, geography, and physical characteristics. As with other characteristics that define people, the meanings of race and ethnicity evolve over time and are subject to a variety of social forces. What it means to be an African American is not acquired innately; it is learned. How these processes unfold has been the focus of racial and ethnic identity development theorists for several decades.

The research of Kenneth and Mamie Clark during the late 1930s and 1940s became a focal point for understanding the psychology of racial identity in black Americans. Their studies of race awareness in black children (Clark and Clark 1939) influenced generations of theorists on racial identity. In their famous doll studies, the Clarks asked children to select either a white or a black doll in response to value-laden commands. Examples of such commands included requests to the children to identify the doll that looked bad, the doll that was a nice color, the doll that looked like the individual child, and the doll that was nice. The researchers demonstrated that black children were able to self-identify accurately and that they showed white preferences consistently (i.e., race dissonance) in their selection of dolls in response to positively valued probes, and black preferences in response to negatively valued probes (Clark and Clark 1947). This race dissonance (i.e., out-group preference) was interpreted as evidence of negative self-esteem and negative self-concept. Indeed, these studies were used as evidence of the psychologically damaging impact of segregation and were prominently referenced in the ruling in favor of Linda Brown in the Supreme Court case *Brown v. Board of Education of Topeka, Kansas* (1954).

Erroneously, race dissonance findings in children were generalized to black adults and to the collective black experience. As a result, a so-called self-hatred hypothesis of black identity found fertile soil and played a prominent role in the theories of social scientists such as Myrdal (1944) and Frazier (1968). The "self-hatred" hypothesis suggested that blacks, as a consequence of their exposure to denigrating and devaluing experiences and stereotypes, internalized negative images of themselves and hence suffered inevitably from low self-esteem.

However, empirical data have illustrated two important phenomena that undermine this hypothesis. First, as research shows, personal and group identities are functionally distinct domains (Cross 1985; Harrison 1985; Krause 1983; Porter and Washington 1979). Second, no significant linearity between race dissonance and self-concept has been found. Margaret Beale Spencer (1982, 1984, 1988) examined the interrelationships among race awareness, race dissonance (white-biased preferences), and self-concept. She interpreted race dissonance among black children as reflective of negative social learning about black people and black things, rather than being feelings they had about themselves. Furthermore, she proposed that there were mediating factors (e.g., church, teachers, family members, community) that cultivated positive self-concepts in most black children, despite their bombardment with negative socialization messages about their race.

The efforts of Thomas (1971) and Cross (1971) were instrumental in fueling inquiry into the nature of black identity and in elucidating the psychology of race and ethnicity. Their efforts, developed in response to the emerging black empowerment movement of the late 1960s and early 1970s, focused on black identity change. Each conceptualized black racial identity as a multistage developmental process that shifted progressively from a negatively charged racial self-concept to a positively charged racial self-concept. Cross (1971, 1991, 1995a) postulated that blacks went through a five-stage process that he called "nigrescence." He named these stages pre-encounter, encounter, immersion/emmersion, internalization, and internalization/commitment. Originally, Cross conceptualized nigrescence as a resocialization process during which blacks moved from "self-hating to self-healing, culturally affirming self-concepts" (Cross 1995b).

More recently, Cross (1991) revised his theory to accommodate research findings showing a continuum of racial attitudes across the racial identity development spectrum, especially in the pre-encounter stage, wherein one can find high racial salience and antiblack attitudes, as well as low salience and neutral attitudes toward blackness. Cross's revisions took into account evidence that blacks in the pre-encounter stage can achieve high self-esteem, even when they attribute low salience to or place low significance on their race or ethnicity. These findings suggested that the individual could develop positive self-regard around some identity aspect other than race. Cross proposed that the construction of a black identity provided the individual with a sense of safety and solidarity.

Parham (1989) introduced the idea of the recycling of the nigrescence process, namely, that even with a traversal through a nigrescence cycle, events or changing circumstances within a person's life may prompt a reworking and reconfiguration of his or her established identity.

These research findings and theories demonstrated immense variability in what race comes to mean to any given individual and further illustrated that self-concept is a function of many personal traits, and not one isolated factor. The findings also illustrate that identity has multiple functions for individuals. Oler (1989) pointed out that there were "different dynamics operating at each stage of Black consciousness development which are central to the Black psyche and can provide useful treatment material for clinicians working with black individuals" (p. 234).

Race and Psychotherapy:
A Brief Overview

Examinations of race and psychotherapy have focused primarily on cross-racial dyads, especially white therapist–black client dyads. Bradshaw (1982) examined the black-white dyad and showed that the white therapist in such a dyad could be influenced by common negative myths and misconceptions about the psychological makeup and social functioning of blacks, including whether they were suitable candidates for psychotherapy. We believe it is also possible for the white therapist to handle race and racial issues adroitly and with minimal bias and misconception.

Little has been written about black-black therapy dyads. However, given the previous discussion on the continuum of racial attitudes among blacks, it is certainly conceivable that black therapists can also hold negative attitudes about blacks, which would undermine the therapeutic process. Indeed, one could argue that any pairing of people, regardless of race, in a therapeutic relationship is fraught with risks for misunderstanding, miscommunication, distrust, and hostility, because all therapists may bring to those relationships divergent experiences and ways of thinking. Hence, every therapeutic dyad may be conceptualized as cross-cultural and capable of poor outcome due to bias and misconception within the therapeutic relationship.

Comas-Diaz and Jacobsen (1991), in their examination of the impact of ethnicity, race, and culture on the psychotherapeutic process, noted a number of ethnocultural transference and countertransference reactions that may aid our understanding of the process. They referred to both *inter*ethnic and *intra*ethnic transference and countertransference reactions that warrant attention and examination in the course of therapy. For example, they described interethnic transference as possibly including overcompliance, denial of differences, and mistrust/hostility. On the other hand, with intraethnic transference, one might see idealization, reaction to the therapist as a traitor or sell-out, or fears of merger. Similarly, countertransferential reactions in an interethnic dyad might include denial of differences, excessive curiosity, or guilt and pity for the disadvantaged. Intraethnic countertransferential reactions might include overidentification and collusion with the patient, or anger that may be aroused because the therapist has not fully processed his or her own feelings and attitudes about racism and discrimination. Comas-Diaz and Jacobsen recommended that therapists be open to understanding both the racial transferences of their clients and their own internal responses to ethnocultural differences, and attend scrupulously to how their internal reactions may affect the treatment relationship.

Rather than focus on race per se, Helms (1990) proposed a racial identity interaction model to facilitate understanding of the impact of race and ethnicity on psychotherapeutic processes. The model has been applied to whites and nonwhites. In Helms's model, "members of all socioracial groups, regardless of specific racial or ethnic group classification, are assumed to experience a racial identity developmental process that can be described by several statuses" (Helms 1995, p. 183). She suggested that differences in racial identity statuses between racial groups could be explained by societal power differential between groups and different socialization experiences. Helms postulated that the racial identity stage or "status" (the term Helms preferred to underscore dynamism rather than stasis) of each participant in a treatment dyad shaped how racial information was processed and understood. Each status has cognitive, affective, and behavioral features that represent how racial material is experienced and processed, and influences racial attitudes and world views. Helms maintained that the locus on the racial identity continuum of each participant in the treatment dyad has profound impact on the treatment relationship.

Helms (1990) described four types of relationships that are a function of these racial identity interactions: parallel, progressive, regressive, and crossed. In *parallel* relationships, the dyadic participants, regardless of race and social power, react to and process racial information in similar ways. In *progressive* relationships, the participant with greater social power interprets and responds to racial events from a more sophisticated status than do participants with lower social power. The dyadic participant having the most social power operates from a more primitive ego status in *regressive* relationships. *Crossed* relationships are those in which the participants perceive and react to racial material in direct opposition to each other.

Carter (1995) undertook research that demonstrated that race alone is not an important variable in psychotherapy, but that racial identity statuses are. He showed that racial identity statuses could vary, could affect the interactions in a dyad, and could influence the therapist's and client's thoughts and behaviors. He used these findings to develop what he called a "Racially Inclusive Model of Psychotherapy."

Carter's and Helms' research and theories were important advances in understanding the complex racial dynamics that operate in psychotherapeutic relationships regardless of the ethnic character or makeup of the dyad's participants.

Case Vignettes

Ms. Jackson

Ms. Jackson is a 55-year-old, divorced, postmenopausal African American woman who was born in a small, rural Southern community, and lived in a three-bedroom house located on the fringes of the inner city. She was employed as a secretarial manager in an academic department at a local university, a job she had held for 20 years. She was married for 15 years prior to her divorce and had three children from that union. Two of her children, both sons, died in their late 20s. One son was a victim of a drive-by shooting; the other died from complications of AIDS. Her daughter, the youngest of her children, shared Ms. Jackson's house, along with the daughter's two young children.

Two months prior to Ms. Jackson's initial consultation, one of her sisters died abruptly of a myocardial infarction. After her sister's death, Ms. Jackson began to visit her internist with increasing frequency because of concerns that something was wrong physically. Her medical complaints consisted primarily of frequent headaches and fatigue. There were no significant medical findings, except for a mild iron-deficiency anemia.

On the day that precipitated her psychiatric referral, Ms. Jackson had visited her doctor's office for a follow-up appointment. The receptionist told her that she would need to find another doctor, because her current doctor was not a participating provider for the health care managed by her new HMO. In a fit of anger, Ms. Jackson became tearful and verbally abusive, and uttered that she wished she were dead. She was then taken to the emergency department and, after evaluation by a psychiatrist, was referred for out-patient follow-up. She requested a black therapist and was, therefore, referred to an African American psychiatrist. Treatment was conducted weekly, over a 5½-month period.

At the time of the initial assessment, Ms. Jackson complained of "bad nerves" and "sleeping problems." During the interview, she described experiencing long-standing "down moods" (even when she was a child). Within the past month, she had found herself becoming increasingly irritable and easily frustrated. She described disturbances of sleep that were characterized by initial and terminal insomnia, as well as early-morning awakening. She suffered poor appetite with significant weight loss, low energy that prompted frequent work absences, poor motivation, a general lack of interest, a feeling of being on the "edge," and poor concentration. A normally neat housekeeper, she reported that her house was "filthy." When she was able to sleep briefly, she often awoke with shortness of breath, a racing heart, and a panicky feeling. She reported having terrible dreams that roused her from sleep, but she could recall no details about them. She denied any active desire to kill herself, although she did express that things sometimes felt so bad she wished "God would take me away." Ms. Jackson denied any previous episodes of this intensity, but she did admit to often "feeling on the down side."

Ms. Jackson revealed that she had been the oldest of three daughters. Her father was the pastor of the largest church in the area. Her mother had worked as a domestic, until her death during childbirth (the child also died) when Ms. Jackson was 8 years old. Within 2 years of her mother's death, Ms. Jackson's father remarried. The stepmother was a teacher who was very strict with the children. Ms. Jackson stated that one could say she grew up in a "middle-class black family."

Tearfully, and with considerable difficulty, Ms. Jackson reported that about 1 month after her mother's death, her father began to fondle her inappropriately ("he touched my privates"), and within 6 months, he had moved to full vaginal penetration of her. Her father had explained to her that it was "just a special love between a father and daughter" and that she must not tell anyone. The sexual abuse continued until Ms. Jackson was 12, the age at which she began her menses. Although she had thought it was wrong, she had never told anyone about it until around 5 years prior to her presentation for therapy, when she told one of her sisters. She made this confession just before her father's death. Ms. Jackson was shocked to discover that her father had also sexually abused her sister. The sister's abuse apparently started after he stopped with Ms. Jackson, and again continued until the sister began her menses. After this sister's death, Ms. Jackson had been thinking "more and more" about the sexual abuse and had had a number of vivid flashbacks.

The therapy with Ms. Jackson was characterized initially by passivity on her part and her expectation that the "doctor" would make her better. She exuded an attitude of helplessness and dependency. She met the diagnostic criteria for dysthymia, major depressive episode, and posttraumatic stress disorder. Within 2 weeks of the start of therapy, Ms. Jackson was started on antidepressant medication, which subsequently proved helpful in ameliorating her depressive symptoms and dampening her anxiety. She continued to experience periodic flashbacks and to be preoccupied about her sister's history of sexual abuse throughout the first 3 months of treatment. Initially, she said very little in the therapy sessions, except to ask how the therapy worked. She was not sure that talking about her life and her past would help, and she felt that it was somewhat damaging to relive the "ugliness of what had happened." She did not believe in her own power to change anything, and she frequently ended a story about her life with the expression, "I guess I'll leave it in the hands of the Lord."

Ms. Jackson was an intelligent woman who sensed that she was burdened by her past. The therapist directed her toward trying to examine why things had worsened so much recently. The therapist pointed out that, despite her many life traumas, she had been functioning quite successfully. Ms. Jackson acknowledged this, and began to talk about how the death of her sister had affected her much harder than she expected. She talked about how she had always tried to keep her emotions in check but had recently found it hard to do. In exploring this aspect of her life, she explained that she never wanted to accept that she needed anything from anyone. This was in contrast to the dependent way in which she responded to the therapist. Indeed, her transference reactions often took on qualities of both neediness and mild flirtatiousness.

Ms. Jackson stated that she had been very close to her mother. Initially, when her father began to visit her in the night, she had enjoyed it and felt comforted in her grief. In the beginning, she said, "He had just held me close like fathers do to their children." As the hugging and touching became more sexual, she was confused, because she knew it was wrong and did not understand why her father thought it was all right. She said, "My father was a preacher, and he should have known it was wrong too. He knew the Bible back and forth."

She confessed a "terrible" thought she had had during the 4 years of abuse, when she would wonder why her father had not chosen one of her sisters. This thought had returned strongly after her sister's death, and each time she thought about it, she felt "heartsick." She reflected that her sister's life had been a "miserable" one and that her sister had suffered bouts of depression and alcoholism, which Ms. Jackson believed were a result of the sexual molestation. She had felt a great deal of guilt and shame when her sister told her that she had also been molested, and wondered if "I had wished this on to her." Ms. Jackson also learned that she had locked away her emotions throughout her life and was able to reflect on how that had affected her relationships.

During the termination of therapy, Ms. Jackson had been surprised by how much she had talked about herself, and she was also surprised that she felt sad, as well as angry, that it was ending. As a result of her openness to these feelings, she was able to reflect on her mother and discovered that her mother's death had evoked both sadness and anger. She recalled being distressed that her mother was having another baby, and she had wished that her mother would not have the baby. This wish became a reality when both her mother and the baby died. Ms. Jackson recalled feeling "horrible" for conjuring up such a thought, and this opened up an examination of her tendency to conceal her wishes and feelings for fear that they would damage, hurt, and destroy. Similarly, the wish that her father would choose one of her sisters came to be understood as her desire for the assaults on her to stop. She became more aware that she was not responsible for her father's behavior or her sister's exploitation by him. By the end of therapy, her depressive symptoms had abated completely, and she no longer had flashbacks or dwelled on her sense of blame about the course of her sister's life. She also found herself better able to express emotions, including anger.

Discussion

This case illustrates the principle that in conducting therapy with African American patients, it is critical to understand that they present with conventional and routine complaints. African Americans undergo depression, anxiety, and trauma. They experience loss, separation, guilt, and shame. They contend with feelings of unworthiness and low self-esteem. And they experience these struggles as a function of being human beings, not as a function of being African Americans. In Ms. Jackson's story, it is the nature of her life that has created her difficulties, not the pigment of her skin or her racial category. Yet there are indeed characteristics of the case that warrant comment with respect to race and ethnicity.

The path to the psychotherapist is rather indirect, and this is common among African Americans who ultimately connect with a mental health professional. Ms. Jackson had been directed to psychological treatment only after she had presented to her internist for more than a month with complaints that could have easily been understood as psychological, once the history was known. Surveys have shown that the help-seeking pathway among African Americans begins frequently with social service agencies or a general medical office (Neighbors 1984, 1985). The stigma of being seen by a psychiatrist or psychologist is often a major impediment to treatment and must be addressed directly. Very often the therapist must be quite active initially to educate the patient about the treatment process and to clarify what the patient is experiencing and expecting. If a diagnosis is made, one should take care to explain clearly what this means and what course of treatment is warranted.

Issues about confidentiality are bound to surface. This can become a significant issue for enrollees in managed-care plans, where the insurer may request clinical information to justify the use of services. For someone who is already somewhat reluctant to be in treatment, this could very well be a major obstacle to continuation of care. An effort must be made to assure the patient about his or her rights to privacy and that the therapist will submit only what is essential to an insurer. Additionally, it may be helpful to review with the patient what one is submitting.

In treating any patient, an important immediate task is the development of a therapeutic alliance, an idea that the two participants in the therapy are collaborating in an attempt to alleviate the patient's distress. That alliance rests on the ability to provide a safe environment for personal disclosure. It requires a setting where the patient will be respected and heard and where it is safe. It requires an understanding that the power differential between therapist and patient will not be abused or misapplied. In Ms. Jackson's case, the power dynamics in therapy were complicated by a history of exploitation, in what was supposed to have been a nurturing and caring relationship. So the therapist needed to attend to the provision of a safe and secure relationship.

Many African American patients who present for therapy confront similar issues of power and autonomy in their relationship with the therapist. It is important for therapists in interethnic treatment arrangements to understand the nature of power dynamics within the society at large, in regard to African Americans, and how those dynamics may influence expectations and fears. Similarly, it is also important for therapists in intergender treatment arrangements to be sensitive to issues of power and autonomy. This is of notable importance for patients who have been victimized sexually and physically. In these instances, the therapist must take care to move at a pace determined by the patient. To press too hard may feel like an intrusion, another violation. The therapist should strive to become what Herman (1992) called a witness to the unfolding terror that the patient may have experienced. In Ms. Jackson's case, her sister had shared the experience and knew the history; therefore, her death had created a void born of their connection to a troubled past. This served to complicate the process of grieving and reawakened Ms. Jackson's feelings that she had played some role in creating her sister's difficult life. In the overall scheme of things, this therapy represented just one small phase of Ms. Jackson's recovery from trauma. It is important to understand that therapists may need to attend to other areas of life where the person feels he or she has been victimized. Sometimes, issues of physical and sexual exploitation can be compounded or exacerbated by experiences of social exploitation, based on race, gender, or another category, wherein one feels socially oppressed. The therapist must be attentive to these possibilities and actively pursue their exploration.

Ms. Jackson's case also illustrates another issue that is frequently a part of therapy with African Americans—namely, the conflict between the psychological intervention and religion or spirituality. Of course, this is not unique to African Americans. Although Ms. Jackson relied on her faith and spirituality for comfort and solace, it was also clear that she had conflicting feelings about it. After all, the instrument of her violation had been a preacher, a "man who could quote the Bible back and forth." This issue is raised not so much to debate the role of spirituality in the healing of people or its effectiveness in comforting. Rather, it is raised to prompt consideration of how spirituality may also provide the framework for one to externalize and to expect that the course of one's life cannot be altered by one's efforts. Indeed, there are many people who believe that the course of their lives is predetermined. As a therapist, it is necessary to investigate the tenacity of such beliefs. It is helpful to try to understand the patient's perspective on where the locus of control lies in their lives.

The initial request for a black therapist deserves comment. The clinician needs to understand what drives such a request. Did Ms. Jackson believe she would be safer, or more comfortable? Did she believe that she would be better understood, or better able to avoid conflicts? While one must respect these kinds of wishes, it is also important to determine explicitly what they represent. Often such requests devolve from a fantasy that some shared identity element, such as gender, race/ethnicity, or sexual affinity, will allow the patient to be understood implicitly by the therapist and obviate the tedious work of telling their personal story. Although race and ethnicity may sometimes facilitate a connection, that connection means very little if the patient and the therapist ignore that they may have had very divergent life experiences, despite sharing some outwardly common feature.

Hence, the therapist, in his or her stance of neutrality, must press the patient to define and clarify his or her experiences of the world, including how race and ethnicity, or another identity element, affect those experiences. In interethnic relationships, the therapist must be careful not to allow his or her curiosity about the ethnic or racial experience of the patient to overshadow the concerns the patient brings to the therapy. Patients may respond to excessive focus on their racial or ethnic experience as an imposition on them to educate the therapist rather than to resolve their own conflicts and distress.

Mr. Robinson

Mr. Robinson is a 25-year-old, single African American man who at the time of his presentation to the clinic was a first-year student in law school at an elite university. He was also pursuing a doctorate degree in history from another institution. He had completed all coursework for the doctorate and had already accomplished considerable research on his dissertation topic. A professor, to whom Mr. Robinson had revealed having serious doubts about his future and feeling completely out of place, referred him for psychotherapy. Mr. Robinson explained that he was in a state of "academic paralysis." He believed that the law school, unlike his graduate program in history, was inflexible. Additionally, he reported sensing "racial" and "economic class" tensions between himself and his classmates. Mr. Robinson was seen in 14 sessions for approximately 3½ months.

Mr. Robinson was born and reared in the South and was the oldest sibling and only male of three children, born to an intact family. His father worked as a janitor in a textile factory, and his mother was an unskilled, seasonal farm laborer. Neither parent had completed school beyond 11th grade. His father was functionally illiterate. Mr. Robinson's younger sisters were 10 and 14 years his junior. Mr. Robinson felt responsible for his sisters and had been one of their primary caretakers since their births. Most of his life, the family had lived in abject poverty. For 7 years, the family did not live in a dwelling that had running water. They always struggled to make ends meet, and they relied on food stamps for groceries. Despite hard work, the family was continually in debt and on the brink of financial chaos.

Despite their lack of formal education, the parents encouraged Mr. Robinson to pursue his education, and they frequently talked about his obtaining a college degree. Mr. Robinson always felt that he needed to be a "model of success." He was a stellar student and graduated at the top of his high school class. Although a number of Ivy League schools had pursued him, he chose to attend one of the historically black colleges. He stated, "I knew I would be able to succeed there." Again he excelled and was convinced by a college mentor to pursue an academic career. Although he respected and wanted to please his mentor, he also felt strongly that he needed to do more to help out the family. Ultimately, he pursued graduate study in history as his mentor had suggested, but also subsequently entered law school. Before applying to law school, he learned of his father's ill health and felt that he needed to pursue a "more sure career sooner rather than later." His girlfriend, who was in the process of completing her studies at the same institution Mr. Robinson had attended previously, also influenced his decision.

At the beginning of therapy, Mr. Robinson often spoke of covert race and class tensions between him and his classmates. He noted how "white" everything was in the law school, and how much this differed from college and graduate school, where he had been surrounded by "brothers and sisters from all over the place," who made him more socially comfortable. He described feeling hesitant to "get to know people" and found himself disclosing little information about himself and his background. He felt that his views were quite different from the opinions expressed by his law school classmates. This was evident from many of the class discussions. He thought that his white classmates had no grasp of the experiences of ethnic minorities in the United States and, as a result, were more than willing to denigrate affirmative action programs that had been designed to "correct historical wrongs." He admitted that he found it difficult at times to sit through these discussions, and sometimes his emotionality prevented him from coherently articulating his thoughts. Under those circumstances, he would develop acute feelings of inadequacy and would feel as if he somehow became "a living argument" against affirmative action. Mr. Robinson was also quite critical of his classmates, including other African Americans, when they discussed economic issues in class. He was confident that his classmates had no conception of the particular difficulties faced by people who "lived paycheck to paycheck in grinding poverty."

As the therapy progressed, however, race and class concerns began to recede, as the therapist guided him to speak more about the particularities of his transition from a predominantly black academic environment to a predominantly white one. Mr. Robinson began to talk more about his lifelong struggles to feel accepted. He acknowledged that he had chosen to attend a historically black university because he feared he would fail if he went to any of the predominantly white colleges that pursued him. He minimized his academic achievements because "those schools just don't stack up to Harvard and Yale." He contemplated the growing distance that he had felt between himself and his family, and talked about how, as his experiences expanded in the world, he had less and less in common with them. He spoke poignantly of their lack of understanding of even the basic demands of college. He described how sad he had felt when he realized that his father could not understand him when he attempted to tell him about his dissertation topic. He recalled that the only time he had seen his father cry was when Mr. Robinson discovered that his father could not read. It was at that moment that his father had told him that he "had to get an education" and that he "had to do it for me." Mr. Robinson recalled vividly his father's shame, and also his own embarrassment when he thought about the poverty of his childhood. He expressed envy of others who were financially better off than his family.

Discussion

In this case example, racial identity conflicts were central to the treatment. Although Mr. Robinson, like Ms. Jackson, entered therapy at the prompting of someone else, it is worth noting here that there are indeed African Americans who seek therapy of their own accord. Mr. Robinson was initially nervous about therapy, stating, "My family believes that anyone seeing a psychiatrist must be crazy." This attitude reflected the stigma that is at times associated with seeing a mental health professional, and the therapist must actively address such concerns. Mr. Robinson and his therapist (a black man) discussed the goals of treatment, and Mr. Robinson stated that he was interested in "working without distractions." He talked freely about what he perceived as racism among his colleagues in the university setting. This seemed to be a function of his identification with the black therapist and his assumption that the two had such experiences in common. While this may often be true, it was nonetheless prudent for the therapist to remain neutral as the story unfolded and to press the patient to portray his own experience. The narrative that one brings to therapy is a function of many things, including a wish to portray oneself in the best light. Consequently, the therapist who agrees with everything that a patient recounts limits the possibility of correcting misperceptions and distortions. The art of listening in therapy involves both hearing what is said and sensing what is not said.

As Mr. Robinson spoke angrily of his perception of racism, it became clearer that his feelings of alienation and marginalization were also rooted in something other than his current situation. Despite his high level of achievement, he also struggled with chronic low self-esteem, conflicts about his self-worth, and insecurity. These were reflected in the way he minimized his educational achievements, in how he devalued the college he attended, in his fears about failing in a predominantly white setting, and in his fear that he would be seen in some stereotypical way. It is critical to recognize that as the patient begins to sort through the feelings that arise from such cognitions, he may be forced to confront elements of racial self-hatred or self-denigration. The therapist should not lose sight of the very real possibility that a person of color does experience racial slights, but the therapist must also help the patient toward insight into what these feelings and concerns represent. In this case, Mr. Robinson's self-concept conflicts were disguised by his focus on being a target of racism and insensitivity. It was clarified that the current environment had simply served to activate Mr. Robinson's own preexisting negative, denigrating thoughts about his blackness. His externalization and projection of the bad parts of himself onto people in his environment were aspects of this self-denigration and served to protect his fragile racial self-concept. With these insights, Mr. Robinson was better able to manage the situation and begin the work of finding more adaptive coping mechanisms.

Further therapeutic exploration revealed that he was struggling with a sense of loss of his status as an academic star when he was in a different and more competitive environment. In the face of new demands upon him to demonstrate competence, he became more focused on his differences from others, including other African Americans. He also became anxious that his designation as a model of success would crumble. The exploration of this area of conflict was made possible because the therapist engaged the patient in looking at the concerns as long-standing issues rather than acute ones. Additionally, Mr. Robinson was engaged in looking at the possibility that factors other than exposure to racism had played a role in his self-doubts and chronic low self-esteem.

The therapist's role is not one of proving or disproving the patient's perceptions. It is one of clarifying whether the concerns about race are a product of actual experiences or represent the patient's attempt to avoid looking at what the experiences arouse in him. Under some circumstances, a focus on race matters and racism is a resistance to examining other hurtful, core psychological issues, such as feelings of abandonment and rejection, conflicts that center on competitiveness, fears of separation and loss, struggles related to autonomy and dependence, and struggles over power and impotence, to name a few (Blue and Gonzalez 1992). The pain of racism is derived in large part from a narcissistic injury inflicted on one's self-concept. In situations where race is a prominent issue, the therapist must respect the patient's perceptions, while insisting that the patient consider other dimensions. If the therapist simply accepts the patient's perceptions and reinforces the patient's worldview, there can be no clarification of the distortions that are often a part of human interactions.

Mr. Robinson's therapist helped him to recognize that his emotionally charged intellectual discourses about race and racism, although valid and important, served to mask other core psychological concerns and protected him from exploring other important themes. As the work of therapy progressed, more about Mr. Robinson's internal struggles and experiences emerged. The initial transference encompassed elements of Mr. Robinson's relationship with his mentor from the historically black college that he had attended. It was manifested by his desire to please the therapist, or more specifically, not to disappoint. He was quite deferential at times, and when this was called into question, he explained it by saying that he was giving the therapist the respect due him. In time, the transference became more definitively paternal, and it was within that context that Mr. Robinson began to understand how much he had been burdened in his life by his wishes to redeem his father's life and to overcome the disappointments he felt about his father. He eventually appreciated that his father's shame at being illiterate, and his own shame about his father, fueled his educational pursuits. He acknowledged the anger he felt at recognizing that he felt his life was not his own. This realization echoed in his recollection of his father telling him that he had to get an education for "me."

Mr. Robinson became more aware of long-standing feelings of marginalization that resulted from the extreme poverty he had experienced and from growing up in a household where he was the educated one and where he was made to take on adult responsibilities from a young age. Much of Mr. Robinson's anxiety resulted from the increasing distance he felt between himself and his family, as his experiences of the world diverged significantly from theirs. This insight helped place in context his feelings of alienation in relation to his classmates, with whom he admittedly had not pursued closer relationships. In this regard, he noted that much of his difficulty arose from projecting some of his own psychological conflicts onto others and reacting as if they were coming from outside of himself. Understanding these conflicts did not eliminate them entirely. However, he was able to overcome his work paralysis and perform better academically. Some of this struggle was expected, in light of the previous discussion in this chapter on the role of recycling in the racial identity development model. As Mr. Robinson enters new environments and has new racial experiences, he will likely undertake additional work to reconfigure his racial attitudes and beliefs.

The growing distance he felt from his family generated much anxiety, because he had to contend with feelings of belonging neither to his own family nor to the environment in which he found himself. This is a struggle that one hears about quite frequently in therapy with African Americans, particularly those occupying the middle socioeconomic class and above. The therapist working with African American patients must be attuned to the multiple influences that determine how each patient sees himself or herself, and must guide patients toward clarifying what is critical to understand about their lives. Mr. Robinson had many developmental tasks ahead, including consolidating his sense of personal and racial identity and finding balance between what he wanted to do in his life and his allegiances to his family. Therapists working with patients who are struggling with racial concerns need to familiarize themselves with racial identity development models, as a way to conceptualize the attitudes, behaviors, and affects that are manifestations of each developmental stage. Furthermore, they must elicit from patients the nature of their racial beliefs about their own particular ethnicity and about others.

Conclusion

This chapter could not possibly address all the significant issues that may arise in the psychotherapeutic treatment of African Americans. The cases and the discussions of them were meant to illustrate a set of principles that may be helpful in this form of cross-racial and trans-ethnic treatment. Foremost among these guiding principles is recognition that African Americans present to the psychotherapeutic enterprise with the same ailments and difficulties as people from other ethnic and racial groups, and that therapists need to familiarize themselves with racial identity development models.

It is recommended that the therapist pay close attention to the therapeutic alliance and work collaboratively with the patient in defining the patient's difficulties and settling on a course of action. It is imperative that the therapist take into account the prevailing power dynamics of the society at large and recognize that some patients, by virtue of their socialization experiences, may have certain fears of subjecting themselves to another's influence and authority. Moreover, the therapist should have an appreciation of the variability of attitudes and beliefs that exist among African Americans, and should become more aware of his or her own racial attitudes and racial identity status. Ultimately, the therapist should recognize that race may sometimes be relatively unimportant in psychotherapy, but that the racial identity stage or status of both participants in the treatment dyad will have a powerful influence on the course of that relationship.

References

Blue HC, Gonzalez CA: The meaning of ethnocultural difference: its impact on and use in the psychotherapeutic process, in New Directions in Mental Health. Edited by Greenfield D. San Francisco, CA, Jossey-Bass, 1992, pp 73–84

Bradshaw WH Jr: Supervision in black and white: race as a factor in supervision, in Applied Supervision in Psychotherapy. Edited by Blumenfield M. New York, Grune & Stratton, 1982, pp 200–220

Brown v Board of Education of Topeka, Kansas, 347 U.S. 483 (1954), footnote 11

Carter RT: The Influence of Race and Racial Identity in Psychotherapy: Toward a Racially Inclusive Model. New York, Wiley, 1995

Clark KB, Clark MP: The development of consciousness of self and the emergence of racial identification in Negro pre-school children. J Soc Psychol 10:591–599, 1939

Clark KB, Clark MP: Emotional factors in racial identification and preference in Negro pre-school children. Journal of Negro Education 19:341–350, 1947

Comas-Diaz L, Jacobsen FM: Ethnocultural transferences and countertransference in the therapeutic dyad. Am J Orthopsychiatry 61:392–402, 1991

Cross WE Jr: The Negro to Black conversion experience. Black World 20:13–27, 1971

Cross WE Jr: Black identity: rediscovering the distinction between personal identity and reference group orientation, in Beginnings: The Social and Affective Development of Black Children. Edited by Spencer MB, Brookins GK, Allen WR. Hillsdale, NJ, Erlbaum, 1985, pp 152–172

Cross WE Jr: Shades of Black. Philadelphia, PA, Temple University Press, 1991

Cross WE Jr: The psychology of nigrescence: revising the Cross model, in Handbook of Multicultural Counseling. Edited by Ponterotto JG. Thousand Oaks, CA, Sage, 1995a, pp 93–122

Cross WE Jr: In search of blackness and afrocentricity: the psychology of black identity change, in Racial and Ethnic Identity: Psychological Development and Creative Expression. Edited by Harris HW, Blue HC, Griffith EEH. New York, Routledge, 1995b, pp 53–72

Frazier GF: On Race Relations. Chicago, IL, University of Chicago Press, 1968

Harrison AO: The black family's socializing environment: self-esteem and ethnic attitudes among black children, in Black Children: Social, Educational, and Parental Environments. Edited by McAdoo HP, McAdoo HL. Beverly Hills, CA, Sage, 1985, pp 174–193

Helms JE: Black and White Racial Identity: Theory, Research, and Practice. Westport, CT, Greenwood Press, 1990

Helms JE: An update of Helms' white and people of color racial identity models, in Handbook of Multicultural Counseling. Edited by Ponterotto JG. Thousand Oaks, CA, Sage, 1995, pp 181–197

Herman JL: Trauma and Recovery: The Aftermath of Violence—From Domestic Abuse to Political Terror. New York, Basic Books, 1992

Krause N: The racial context of black self-esteem. Social Psychology Quarterly 46:98–107, 1983

Myrdal G: An American Dilemma: the Negro Problem and Modern Democracy. New York, Harper & Brothers, 1944

Neighbors HW: Professional help use among Black Americans: implications for unmet need. Am J Community Psychol 12:551–566, 1984

Neighbors HW: Seeking professional help for personal problems: Black Americans' use of health and mental health services. Community Ment Health J 21:156–166, 1985

Oler CH: Psychotherapy with Black clients' racial identity and locus of control. Psychotherapy 26:233–241, 1989

Parham TA: Cycles of psychological nigrescence. Counseling Psychologist 17:187–226, 1989

Porter JR, Washington RE: Black identity and self-esteem: a review of studies of black self-concept. Annual Review of Sociology 5:53–74, 1979

Spencer MB: Pre-school children's social cognition and cultural cognition: a cognitive developmental interpretation of race dissonance findings. J Psychol 112:275–296, 1982

Spencer MB: Black children's race awareness, racial attitudes, and self-concept: a reinterpretation. J Child Psychol Psychiatry 25:433–441, 1984

Spencer MB: Self-concept development, in Perspectives in Black Child Development. Edited by Slaughter DT. San Francisco, CA, Jossey-Bass, 1988, pp 59–72

Thomas CW: Boys No More. Beverly Hills, CA, Glencoe, 1971

CHAPTER 11

The Hispanic Veteran

Jose M. Cañive, M.D.
Diane T. Castillo, Ph.D.
Vicente B. Tuason, M.D.

In this chapter, we offer several case vignettes to illustrate the impact of cultural issues in the therapy of male and female Hispanic veterans. Four cases are briefly described, two males and two females; the identities of the patients have been disguised. In three of the cases, the patient carries a diagnosis of posttraumatic stress disorder (PTSD). A discussion section, where the specific cultural aspects of treatment are elaborated, follows each case presentation. We then provide an overview of traditional Hispanic culture in order to emphasize its most salient features: language, familism, and spirituality. We conclude the chapter with a discussion of frequently encountered themes in the treatment of Hispanic veterans, including self-disclosure, cultural explanations of illness, and cultural validity of standardized psychological assessment instruments.

Case Vignettes

Mr. Rodríguez

Mr. Rodríguez, a 61-year-old, married, Hispanic veteran of the Korean War, sought treatment for his combat-related PTSD from a structured Veterans Administration (VA) PTSD program. Initial assessment interviews were conducted by different team clinicians before the patient was accepted into the treatment program. The program offered a cognitive-behavioral therapeutic orientation and emphasized treatment exposure. He was assigned a younger African American woman as primary therapist. Early in treatment, the assigned therapist identified the patient as resistant to exposure therapy because he refused to disclose details of his war traumas, an essential component of that treatment modality. At the weekly staff meeting, it became obvious that the patient had discussed the details of his traumas with the Hispanic male staff, who gathered the military history during assessment. Mr. Rodríguez's reassignment to the Hispanic male staff, who obtained the military history, led to successful therapy engagement and completion of intensive treatment. As part of his aftercare treatment, he was assigned a Hispanic female therapist. He established a lasting therapeutic alliance with her and continues to see her periodically on the anniversary dates of his traumas. Over a period of 7 years, he has been able to reveal to her the most intimate details of his traumatic events.

Discussion

Several cultural issues become evident in this case: self-disclosure, therapist gender, and development of *confianza* (rapport, trust). The first and most important is the patient's inability to discuss his war traumas with the therapist. Traditional Hispanic males may be extremely concerned about the "fragility" of females and feel the need to protect them from listening to narratives about grotesque, disgusting, and inhuman war events. Mr. Rodríguez did not worry about disclosing his traumas to a male therapist, but he could not bring himself to reveal the revolting events to a female. As a child, he had learned that females could not tolerate *emociones fuertes* (strong emotions) and that it was his duty as a male to shelter them from such emotions. He may have heard that women, more often than men, may die of *susto* (fright) following an intense emotional event. Mr. Rodríguez truly believed that disclosing the details of his war trauma (killing a civilian woman) to a female therapist might ultimately cause her death.

Another important factor that may have interfered with disclosure was shame. The strong traditional Catholic orientation of most Hispanics, with its emphasis on the Virgin Mary, may have augmented Mr. Rodríguez's shame of killing a woman. Women, as replicas of the Virgin Mary, are perceived as pure and innocent. Thus, killing an innocent woman may have the connotation of killing Mary, a horrendous crime.

Further obstacles to self-disclosure included traditional Hispanics' attitudes, which discourage sharing intimate emotional problems with strangers (i.e., people outside the immediate family). Years of interpersonal contact with a female Hispanic therapist eventually allowed Mr. Rodríguez to develop the needed *confianza* to overcome his reticence to share his traumatic events with a woman and to get closer to his own self-forgiveness.

Related themes in this case are the possible advantages and disadvantages of a therapist and patient having the same ethnic background, and the perils of intercultural psychotherapy. A therapist of the same ethnic background as the patient may establish immediate rapport (Westermeyer 1989), since a common cultural heritage will enhance the patient's perception of an empathic and competent therapist (Nguyen 1992). Hispanic therapists may intuitively behave with *personalismo,* the personal touch and small informality demanded of professionals in Hispanic cultures (Acosta and Evans 1982; Martínez 1993), increasing the patient's level of comfort and desire to share his or her intimate problems. On the other hand, Hispanic therapists may feel overconfident and may not recognize the import of education and social class differences (Martínez 1993). Moreover, therapists from the same ethnic background may fail to explore deep underlying issues, since they may identify with the patient (cultural countertransference) and may be easily sidetracked by the patient's prominent cultural symptoms (Nguyen 1992). This concept of *cultural countertransference* (Spiegel 1976; Westermeyer 1989) is also of great importance for therapists of other ethnic backgrounds, since the feelings and attitudes of a therapist toward a patient's culture may have an impact on the clinical encounter. Psychotherapy education, training, and supervision are key to dealing with these issues.

Mr. García

Mr. García, a 55-year-old married, Hispanic veteran, presented for treatment with multiple somatic complaints. Since his combat experience in Vietnam, he had never sought help from mental health care providers. He spontaneously reported back pain, dizziness, chest pain, and difficulty breathing. Only on further inquiry did the symptoms of depression and PTSD become evident. He apologized for seeking help and for taking time from the clinician. Once a therapeutic alliance was established, he developed an excellent relationship with a Hispanic psychiatrist and responded well to psychopharmacological and cognitive-behavioral therapy interventions.

Discussion

Mr. García demonstrated commonly held attitudes of Hispanic patients about mental health care. First, he was not psychologically minded and felt unworthy of treatment. Psychological distress is revealed through somatic complaints, which are mostly reported to the family physician and are seldom the basis for referral to mental health specialists. Feeling unworthy of treatment and embracing the attitude of *lo que Dios quiera* (whatever God wills) fed into his pattern of untreated chronic psychiatric symptoms. In addition, Hispanics and other minorities are often unaware of available community mental health services, and this decreases their likelihood of obtaining treatment. Moreover, Mr. García also attributed his illnesses to preternatural causes. *Lo que Dios quiera* means that illnesses are given and taken away by special powers beyond the person's control. This belief may foster feelings of powerlessness, decreased self-esteem, and perception of the doctor as a powerful, God-sent being. Therefore, the patient may be wrongly perceived as an extremely passive agent in therapy. Gender issues also contributed to these attitudes, since Mr. García believed that complaining is not for men.

Once a therapeutic alliance was established, he developed a clear psychological understanding of the emotional forces that partially accounted for his current emotional condition. In other words, he became more psychologically minded and was able to generate not only compassion but also professional satisfaction from the therapist. His exemplary compliance with treatment, and his enthusiastic expressions of gratefulness, helped the therapist re-evaluate his initial negative countertransference and perception of the patient as dependent and unmotivated. Parenthetically, Hispanic patients with this constellation of symptoms and help-seeking attitudes often seek the services of *curanderos* (traditional cultural healers), frequently with successful outcomes.

Ms. Garduño

Ms. Garduño is a 31-year-old, Hispanic Gulf War veteran with PTSD who resided in a rural community, approximately 150 miles from the VA hospital. She lived with her female partner and her partner's 8-year-old daughter. She described having a close relationship with her mother, and her apartment was a short distance from the parental home. Although the mother and other family members were aware of the lesbian relationship, the subject was never openly discussed. Ms. Garduño was Catholic and often referred to God and the Bible as her source of strength and inspiration. She sought treatment after being incarcerated because of a violent argument with her partner. During assessment, she reported childhood sexual abuse by an uncle but denied any emotional difficulties related to the abuse. She emphasized feeling safe, since immediately after informing her parents, her uncle was expelled from the household and further abuse was prevented. At the beginning of treatment, she complied with scheduled appointments and attended regularly the time-demanding (3 days a week), structured treatment program. After unsuccessful outpatient treatment, she was referred to an inpatient treatment program located out of the state. Upon her return to New Mexico, she was assigned to an aftercare group and to a female Hispanic therapist for individual treatment. Although she initially attended sessions regularly, her attendance eventually dropped off. She continued to seek help from her therapist during crises and attended medication management sessions with a psychiatrist.

Discussion

The issues that emerge in the case of Ms. Garduño include treatment engagement, therapy expectations, self-disclosure, and gender roles. Although Ms. Garduño appeared involved in treatment at each stage of the process, she never fully engaged in therapy. Her reticence to disclose sensitive information could be attributed to the common resistance to therapy encountered with PTSD patients. However, cultural factors most likely contributed to her resistance. Most traditional Hispanics maintain that emotional pain, particularly if attached to potential sources of embarrassment, should be discussed only with family members. It is of interest that Ms. Garduño was able to disclose the details of her childhood sexual molestation but was incapable of discussing her war traumas in depth. This apparent contradiction is elucidated by the way her family handled her childhood sexual molestation. Upon learning about the events, her parents immediately confronted and barred the uncle from the household. She was present during the confrontation and felt protected, loved, and reassured. Although only speculative, it is quite possible that the early resolution of her sexual trauma accounted for the ease of her disclosure. On the other hand, witnessing the deaths of friends and civilians during the Gulf War occurred away from home and violated cultural-religious values about the reverence for life. Her inability to fully engage in treatment and work through her combat trauma could be related to her expectations of an immediate resolution, similar to the resolution of her sexual trauma. Working through the combat trauma was impeded immediately by the geographical distance from her family and, later, by the lack of family context in the treatment setting.

Another important issue in this case is the family members' acceptance of her sexual orientation. In traditional Hispanic culture, gender roles are clearly stipulated, and people are socially ostracized for deviation from their roles. Although these attitudes change according to acculturation and epoch, Ms. Garduño lived within a traditional family in a small Hispanic town. The mother's acceptance of Ms. Garduño's sexual orientation seemed to be based on fear of losing *mi hijita* (my special little daughter), but she seemed to be unable to reconcile her values with her daughter's sexual orientation. As a result, the mother, while caring and overprotective, was emotionally unavailable during her daughter's stressful experiences with her partner. The dynamics of the mother-daughter relationship, along with the patient's PTSD hyperarousal symptoms, may explain why her frequent emotional crises led to hospitalization and even incarceration. To date, Ms. Garduño's combat trauma has not been properly addressed, since interruptions in treatment have been the rule. Missing in her treatment approach has been family involvement. Family members might have become powerful allies in treatment by providing the emotional context necessary to arrive at the successful resolution of Ms. Garduño's war traumas.

Ms. Gómez

The director of the general outpatient clinic referred Ms. Gómez, a 59-year-old, divorced, Hispanic veteran, to a Hispanic female therapist. She had dropped out of treatment with a Caucasian male therapist and requested assignment to "a woman therapist who can understand my feelings better." She presented with symptoms of depression and anxiety and stated that her treatment goal was to prevent another episode of depression.

Ms. Gómez's first depressive episode had occurred 11 years before this clinical encounter. She had once suffered from alcoholism but had been abstinent from alcohol for 21 years and had been attending weekly Alcoholics Anonymous (AA) meetings throughout her sobriety. She had an older and a younger brother who lived on her parents' farm. Ms. Gómez, on the other hand, lived in a city 60 miles away from the parental household. As her parents aged, she steadily assumed greater responsibilities for her ailing father's care, whom she perceived as being neglected by her mother and brothers.

She spent 3 days a week at the parent's home in order to properly feed, bathe, and help her father with physical exercise. Since this arrangement did not work out to her satisfaction, she brought her father to live with her, and as his medical needs increased, she placed him in a retirement home. Still unsatisfied with his care, she took him back to his farm, after installing her trailer on the farm, in close proximity to the parental household. She stopped participating in all social activities, with the exception of weekly AA meetings. Ms. Gómez perceived the relationship with her mother as extremely stressful, since the mother continually criticized her actions. Ms. Gómez's contact with her only daughter was limited to providing baby-sitting services for her granddaughter in the city during her few hours away from her father.

Discussion

This case illustrates the traditional role of *la sufrida* (the suffering woman), often assumed by single or divorced women in traditional Hispanic families (Bach-y-Rita 1982). Ms. Gómez appears to be caught in that role to the detriment of her own mental health. The pivotal role of the family in the lives of almost all individuals of Hispanic origin has been emphasized by a number of authors (Escobar and Randolph 1982; Koss-Chioino and Cañive 1996; Murillo 1971). Traditional Hispanics perceive their families as a "major source of strength" and "their fountain of comfort" (Murillo 1971), although the Hispanic family has also been described as a "double-edged sword" (Keefe et al. 1979). In spite of two married male siblings who lived on the parents' farm, Ms. Gómez returned home to take care of her ailing father. Her brothers, as male children, felt less obliged to nurse their ailing father, and they colluded by assigning their sister the role of caretaker. The demands of the assigned role interfered with Ms. Gómez's involvement in activities that could bring her personal satisfaction or nourish her emotional well-being. She appeared obsessed about ensuring her father's well-being and felt content being her father's caregiver. She neglected her physical and psychological needs, as well as the needs of her own immediate family. She was raised in an extended family, moved into her own nuclear family, but eventually took on the major responsibilities of her family of origin. Ms. Gómez accepted her role graciously, with no complaints. The role is culturally prescribed, and, like many other women in traditional Hispanic society, she knew it was "the right thing to do."

The first therapist identified the family obligations as the main source of her depression and confronted the patient with his perception. This therapeutic approach did not yield results, as Ms. Gómez angrily withdrew from treatment. The therapist did not recognize the import of the patient's culturally prescribed role and alienated her from therapy with his suggestions. Ms. Gómez felt misunderstood, since it seemed inconceivable that somebody would suggest she should abandon her ailing father. Thus, she requested a female therapist capable of understanding her predicament. The second therapist, a Hispanic female, was better acquainted with the role of women in Hispanic families. The therapist empathized with Ms. Gómez's family situation, through sharing her own experiences with the patient. The therapist also underlined the difficulties younger women face keeping up with the customs and expectations of the older generation. Ms. Gómez looked forward to the therapy sessions and started paying more attention to her own personal needs. The patient was also able to switch from English to Spanish during the sessions and felt the therapist understood the true meaning of her emotions, because she could not convey her emotions well in the English language.

Salient Features of
Hispanic Culture

Culture refers to the customs, shared beliefs, and social organization of a people. In a more colloquial way, and paraphrasing Bock (1970), culture is what makes us strangers in a foreign country. It is what constitutes people's world of meanings. Hispanics' worldviews derive from three main sources: Spain, North and South America (among native groups), and Africa (mostly from the Yoruba tribe, today's South Nigeria) (Ramirez 1991). Differences in worldviews are increased by a number of factors, among them, patterns of migration, age at migration, level of acculturation, socioeconomic status, education, and occupation (Rosado and Elias 1993). Despite the heterogeneity of Hispanic minorities in the United States, there are similarities in the organizations of their local worlds. Language, familism, and spirituality are facets of Hispanic culture that may affect the clinical encounter.

Language

Community studies found that 70%–83% of Hispanics preferred to be interviewed in Spanish (Lang et al. 1982). Furthermore, 47% of the Mexican American respondents to the National Institute of Mental Health (NIMH) Epidemiologic Catchment Area (ECA) survey completed the interview in

Spanish (Karno 1994). Several studies have shown that Spanish-speaking patients with limited English proficiency are rated as having a higher severity of psychopathology when interviewed in English (Marcos et al. 1973). The patient's general attitude toward the clinician, motor activity, speech, affect, and sense of self are strongly influenced by the language barrier.

Another important aspect of language in the treatment of Hispanic patients is the frequent use of code (language) switching. Hispanic veterans often abruptly switch from English to Spanish when anxious or when expressing strong emotions. In other instances, code switching may be used as a defensive maneuver to alienate the therapist from understanding the patient's psychiatric difficulties (Marcos 1976). This language switching not only annoys the unaware clinician but also may make the patient's speech appear confused and his or her thinking illogical. Therapists must be attentive, since switching language during a session often carries a powerful message, not to be ignored (Russell 1988).

Familism

Another common characteristic of Hispanic culture is the reliance of the individual on the family. Marin and Van Oss Marin (1991) include under the characteristic *familism* three types of value orientations: 1) family members are expected to provide material and emotional support to one another, 2) they expect to rely on other family members for such support, and 3) they look to relatives to model proper conduct and good attitudes. In the clinic setting, this family interdependence may be interpreted as a sign of lack of motivation for treatment when the patient expresses the need to consult with his or her family before making a treatment decision (Koss-Chioino and Cañive 1996). Similarly, Hispanic veterans who are living with their elderly parents may be labeled as dependent and weak, when they are, in fact, adhering to traditional family values. Canceling of appointments to attend family functions appears unjustified and is often interpreted as resistance to treatment, unless the values inherent to an extended family system are considered.

Mothers, worried about the suffering of *mi hijito* (my baby), may inadvertently enable their sons in self-medication addiction or sabotage treatment efforts. This family overinvolvement, when not managed appropriately, can be a hindrance to treatment; however, the benefits of unconditional family support cannot be ignored. Educating and involving parents and significant extended family members in treatment decisions, if not in therapy, is of great clinical import.

Spirituality

Most Hispanics value *spirituality,* defined as a sense of wholeness, inner peace, interconnection, and reverence for life (Cervantes and Ramirez 1992). These values may be expressed through organized religion and belief in a higher power, particularly through Roman Catholicism, but are also expressed through personal ideologies and folk religions. Spirituality summarizes the ideals that family life must fulfill. The clinical relevance of this religious orientation can be seen in the impact that numerous Catholic rituals have throughout the life cycle: baptism, confirmation, First Holy Communion, marriage, and death. These religious events are occasions to strengthen family relationships and to extend family boundaries by including close friends, in the role of *compadres,* within the "bosom of the family."

Outside the Catholic religion, Hispanics often express their beliefs in a higher power through their reliance on folk healers (*curanderos* among Mexican Americans, spiritualists among Puerto Ricans, and *santeras* among Cuban Americans). These traditional healers represent the fusion of American Indian or African spiritual beliefs with Catholic faith. Hispanic veterans often seek the support and remedies of *curanderas,* although they seldom reveal this to their therapists. Their strong cultural-spiritual orientation has led therapists to encourage specific spiritual practices, such as lighting candles to the saints during trauma anniversaries. Treatment programs often include quasi-spiritual rituals in their treatment. For example, veterans are led on a pilgrimage to a nearby war memorial, where they light candles and read letters pregnant with emotions about their traumas. At the end of the ceremony, the letters are burned, an act that symbolizes the cleansing of their inner beings.

Assessment Issues

Among many issues cited in the literature, it seems particularly important to address the following when evaluating and treating Hispanic veterans: self-disclosure, idioms of distress, and the cultural validity of structured interviews, self-rating scales, and psychological tests.

Self-Disclosure

Traditional Hispanic cultures socialize the individual to confide in family members and to not disclose intimate emotional problems to strangers (Koss-Chioino and Cañive 1996). In addition, men learn that issues and concerns related to sex and aggression should not be discussed with women. Therefore, veterans' common reticence to disclose details of their military history is heightened among Hispanics. A longer period of time to establish *confianza* (trust) is required prior to disclosure of traumatic events (Rosado and Elias 1993). Moreover, Hispanic veterans often will not disclose significant details of their traumas to women therapists because of shame and, perhaps more important, factors related to traditional Hispanic male socialization patterns, which emphasize their gender superiority and their responsibilities as financial and emotional providers and protectors of family members, especially women.

Culturally Determined Idioms of Distress

Conceptions of illness and symptom expression are culturally bound (Hughes 1993). Hispanic veterans with PTSD may express their symptoms and social support needs through a number of idioms of distress. Perhaps the most common idiom of distress used by Hispanics is *somatization* (Escobar et al. 1987, 1992; Kleinman 1986). Hispanic veterans often present with a variety of somatic complaints, sometimes masking their PTSD symptoms and raising questions about their correct diagnosis. Another frequently used idiom of distress is *nervios* (Jenkins 1988), a state of vulnerability to stress characterized by irritability, inability to concentrate, and dizziness, among other symptoms.

Hispanic patients often seek illness explanations in the supernatural. For example, it is not uncommon for Hispanics to attribute their illness to *susto,* a frightening event that causes the soul to separate from the body (Rubel 1964). Similarly, being hexed, or *embrujado,* serves to explain a wide variety of symptoms (Koss-Chioino and Cañive 1993). Patients seldom reveal their explanatory models of illness spontaneously; instead, these models need to be elicited by the clinician. Understanding the patient's idioms of distress and explanatory models may be crucial to arriving at a correct diagnosis and establishing a therapeutic relationship, which includes the patient's conception of the clinical reality.

Cross-Cultural Validity of Assessment Measures

No assessment measure or psychological test is absolutely culture free (Westermeyer 1993). Standardization of PTSD structured interviews and self-rating scales with Hispanic populations is sorely needed, since most measures have been developed in Anglo society, with a theoretical base anchored in a Western viewpoint of psychopathology. Further, idioms of distress and conceptions of illness frequently invoked by Hispanics are not included in the existing questionnaires (Marsella et al. 1993). Ethnic minorities score higher (indicating more pathology) on several scales of the Minnesota Multiphasic Personality Inventory (MMPI) (Gynther 1972). However, retrospective data from our clinic revealed no significant differences between Anglos and Hispanics on the MMPI-2, except for attenuated PTSD scale scores among Hispanics with current alcohol abuse (Weaver et al. 1995). Nonetheless, conclusions made with measures that have not been culturally validated should be interpreted with caution.

Following Hinton and Kleinman (1993), we propose the following guidelines to arrive at diagnosis and a culturally appropriate formulation:

1. Be empathetic from the beginning, and elicit the veteran's ideas about his or her suffering.
2. Assess the patient's illness experience within his or her sociocultural context: family, work, health care system, local community.
3. Arrive at a diagnosis by using not only DSM-IV (American Psychiatric Association 1994) categories but the veteran's cultural idioms of distress as well. Additionally, it is paramount that the team of clinicians reach a consensus about the diagnosis.

Treatment Considerations

Crisis Orientation

Hispanics tend to seek services during crisis periods and may not follow through with treatment. This crisis orientation does not represent resistance to treatment; rather, it may be related to socioeconomic difficulties (Rosado and Elias 1993) and, in the case of Hispanic males, the belief that seeking help denotes weakness. It must also be noted that, typically, less-acculturated Hispanics are not psychologically minded (Acosta and Evans 1982). This common problem may be partially addressed through patient and family education and assertive case follow-up, by which the hope is to establish a therapeutic alliance. A more comprehensive approach would include the development of alternative treatment strategies that are more compatible with Hispanics' worldview and socioecological realities (Rogler et al. 1987).

Direct Advice

The scientific literature also describes Hispanics as being more amenable to advice and counsel than to insight-oriented therapy. Thus, cognitive and behavioral therapies, which provide specific instructions on "how to," may be better suited than individual insight-oriented psychotherapy for this population. One caveat of this approach is that patients may passively go along with what the therapist suggests, since unquestioned acceptance of authority is a traditional value among Hispanics. Therefore, therapists need to encourage patients to express disagreement (Acosta and Evans 1982).

Negotiation of Explanatory Models

Therapists need to negotiate treatment with their veterans on the basis of the explanatory models to which veterans and their families adhere. It is useless to make patients develop our insight and adhere to our "scientific" conceptions of illness, when they have been socialized to believe that their illnesses may be caused by being *embrujado* (hexed), suffering from *susto,* or being punished for their sins. Instead, it is important to elicit and respect their beliefs, while describing our professional explanatory models and openly considering referral to religious authorities and folk healers, if deemed appropriate. Premature treatment termination and lack of treatment compliance are often the result of this lack of understanding.

Cultural Adaptation of Program Content and Context

Service models are often based on premises that may be invalid in other cultures and that, therefore, may require adaptations of their format and content. Mental health professionals, often unaware of popular conceptions of mental illness, may believe that individual independence is the gold standard of therapy and that mental health services are provided equally to everyone. They may not realize that there is life beyond the nuclear family and that rules of effective communication and strategies for problem solving are not universal. Understanding these false assumptions will lead therapists to modify their approaches and to develop more culturally sensitive interventions.

The service delivery format can be enhanced through providing a casual clinic atmosphere and including extended family members in treatment. In general, mental health professionals should be more emotionally responsive to ensure therapeutic engagement. Showing Hispanic veterans *respeto* (respect), *dignidad* (dignity), and *cariño* (caring) is essential to the therapeutic process.

Similarly, adaptation of treatment program content needs to be considered. For example, folk explanations of illness should be discussed during the psychoeducational phase of treatment. Family overinvolvement may be

reframed as devoted concern for the patient, and not labeled as enmeshment. Powerful metaphors to use in therapy may be found in often colloqui-
ally used Spanish sayings or proverbs (*dichos o refranes*) (Zuniga 1992).
Also, commonly used skill training modules should be scrutinized and
adapted for use with Hispanic veterans. Finally, it is recommended that therapists engage in simple cultural sensitivity exercises, such as those proposed
by Pinderhughes (1989), to increase awareness of their cultural heritage and
to better understand cultural differences.

Conclusion

Providing therapy to Hispanic veterans brings closer to home many of the
cultural issues encountered in the treatment of Hispanic minorities. Common occurrences in military service include racial discrimination, combat
exposure, and long-lasting emotional reactions to human violence and trauma. These experiences exquisitely increase the sensitivity of Hispanic veterans to feeling used, unheard, misunderstood, and mistreated. Therapists
need to be ever more knowledgeable about the veterans' cultural beliefs, values, and attitudes. The patients' raw anger, covered up emotions, and pro-
tective defenses may constantly test therapists' emotions and skills. Finally,
the heterogeneity of Hispanics should be strongly emphasized, since general
descriptors about Hispanics have been discussed, and cultural stereotyping
is to be avoided. The information presented here should be only the prelude
to formulating and testing hypotheses in actual clinical work.

References

Acosta FX, Evans LA: The Hispanic-American patient, in Effective Psychotherapy for
    Low-Income and Minority Patients. Edited by Acosta FX, Yamamoto J, Evans
    LA. New York, Plenum, 1982, pp 51–82
American Psychiatric Association: Diagnostic and Statistical Manual of Mental Dis-
    orders, 4th Edition. Washington, DC, American Psychiatric Association, 1994
Bach-y-Rita G: The Mexican American: religious and cultural influences, in Mental
    Health and Hispanic Americans: Clinical Perspectives. Edited by Becerra R, Karno
    M, Escobar J. New York, Grune & Stratton, 1982, pp 29–40
Bock PK: Culture Shock: A Reader in Modern Cultural Anthropology. New York,
    Knopf, 1970
Cervantes JM, Ramirez O: Spirituality and family dynamics in psychotherapy with
    Latino children, in Working With Culture: Psychotherapeutic Interventions With

Ethnic Minority Children and Adolescents. Edited by Vargas LA, Koss-Chioino JD. San Francisco, CA, Jossey-Bass, 1992, pp 103–128

Escobar JI, Randolph ET: The Hispanic and social networks, in Mental Health and Hispanic Americans: Clinical Perspectives. Edited by Becerra R, Karno M, Escobar J. New York, Grune & Stratton, 1982, pp 41–57

Escobar JI, Burman A, Karno M: Somatization in the community. Arch Gen Psychiatry 44:713–718, 1987

Escobar JI, Canino G, Rubio-Stipec M: Somatic symptoms after a natural disaster: a prospective study. Am J Psychiatry 149:965–967, 1992

Gynther MB: White norms and black MMPIs: a prescription for discrimination? Psychol Bull 78:386–402, 1972

Hinton L IV, Kleinman A: Cultural issues and international psychiatric diagnosis, in International Review of Psychiatry. Edited by Costa e Silva JA, Nadelson CC. Washington, DC, American Psychiatric Press, 1993, pp 111–129

Hughes CC: Culture in clinical psychiatry, in Culture, Ethnicity, and Mental Illness. Edited by Gaw AC. Washington, DC, American Psychiatric Press, 1993, pp 3–42

Jenkins JH: Ethnopsychiatric interpretations of schizophrenic illness: the problem of nervios within Mexican American families. Cult Med Psychiatry 12:301–329, 1988

Karno M: The prevalence of mental disorder among persons of Mexican birth and origin, in Latino Mental Health: Current Research and Policy Perspectives. Edited by Telles C, Karno M. Washington, DC, U.S. Department of Health and Human Services, 1994, pp 3–16

Keefe SE, Padilla AM, Carlos MI: The Mexican American extended family as an emotional support system. Real and extended familism among Mexican Americans and Anglo Americans: on the meaning of code family ties. Human Organization 38:144–152, 1979

Kleinman A: Social Origins of Distress and Disease. New Haven, CT, Yale University Press, 1986

Koss-Chioino JD, Cañive JM: The interaction of cultural and clinical diagnostic labeling: the case of embrujado. Med Anthropol 15:171–188, 1993

Koss-Chioino JD, Cañive JM: Cultural issues in relational diagnosis: Hispanics in the United States, in Handbook of Relational Diagnosis and Dysfunctional Family Patterns. Edited by Kaslow FW. New York, Wiley, 1996, pp 137–151

Lang JG, Munoz RF, Bernal G, et al: Quality of life and psychological well-being in a bicultural Latino community. Hispanic Journal of Behavioral Science 4:433–445, 1982

Marcos L: Bilinguals in psychotherapy: language as an emotional barrier. Am J Psychother 30:552–560, 1976

Marcos LR, Alpert M, Urcuyo L, et al: The effect of interview language on the evaluation of psychopathology I: Spanish-American schizophrenic patients. Am J Psychiatry 130:549–553, 1973

Marin G, Van Oss Marin B: Research With Hispanic Populations (Applied Social Research Method Series Vol 23). London, Sage, 1991

Marsella AJ, Friedman MJ, Spain EH: Ethnocultural aspects of posttraumatic stress disorder, in American Psychiatric Press Review of Psychiatry, Vol 12. Edited by Oldham JM, Riba MB, Tasman A. Washington, DC, American Psychiatric Press, 1993, pp 157–181

Martínez C: Psychiatric care of Mexican Americans, in Culture, Ethnicity, and Mental Illness. Edited by Gaw AC. Washington, DC, American Psychiatric Press, 1993, pp 431–466

Murillo N: The Mexican American family, in Chican: Social and Psychological Perspectives. Edited by Hernandez CA, Huang MJ, Wagner NN. St Louis, MO, CV Mosby, 1971, pp 155–170

Nguyen NA: Living between two cultures: treating first-generation Asian Americans, in Working With Culture: Psychotherapeutic Interventions With Ethnic Minority Children and Adolescents. Edited by Vargas LA, Koss-Chioino JD. San Francisco, CA, Jossey-Bass, 1992, pp 204–222

Pinderhughes E: Understanding Race, Ethnicity, and Power: The Key to Efficacy in Clinical Practice. New York, Free Press, 1989

Ramirez M: Psychotherapy and Counseling With Minorities: A Cognitive Approach to Individual and Cultural Differences. New York, Pergamon, 1991

Rogler LH, Malgady RG, Constantino G, et al: What do culturally-sensitive mental health services mean? The case of Hispanics. Am Psychol 42:565–570, 1987

Rosado JW Jr, Elias MJ: Ecological and psychocultural mediators in the delivery of services for urban, culturally diverse Hispanic clients. Professional Psychology: Research and Practice 24:450–459, 1993

Rubel A: The epidemiology of a folk illness: susto in Hispanic America. Ethnology 3:268–283, 1964

Russell DM: Language and psychotherapy: the influence of non-standard English in clinical practice, in Clinical Guidelines in Cross-Cultural Mental Health. Edited by Comas-Díaz L, Griffith EEH. New York, Wiley, 1988, pp 126–136

Spiegel JP: Cultural aspects of transference and countertransference revisited. J Am Acad Psychoanal 4:447–467, 1976

Weaver DD, Castillo DT, Howard RA, et al: MMPI-2 profiles of Hispanic Vietnam combat veterans. Poster presented at the annual meeting of the International Society for Traumatic Stress Studies, Chicago, November 1995

Westermeyer JJ: The Psychiatric Care of Migrants: A Clinical Guide. Washington, DC, American Psychiatric Press, 1989

Westermeyer JJ: Cross-cultural psychiatric assessment, in Culture, Ethnicity, and Mental Illness. Edited by Gaw AC. Washington, DC, American Psychiatric Press, 1993, pp 125–144

Zuniga ME: Using metaphors in therapy: Dichos and Latino clients. Soc Work 37:55–60, 1992

CHAPTER 12

The Southeast Asian Refugee: The Legacy of Severe Trauma

J. David Kinzie, M.D.

T he Vietnam War resulted in 700,000 refugees from Vietnam, Cambodia, and Laos (Mollica 1994). Studies of these refugees were initiated soon after they began arriving in the United States in 1975. In the early studies, depression was found to be common (Kinzie and Manson 1983). However, after the introduction of DSM-III in 1980 (American Psychiatric Association 1980), in which the diagnosis of posttraumatic stress disorder (PTSD) was identified with specific criteria, PTSD was found to be the most important condition in clinical populations (Boehnlein et al. 1985; Kinzie et al. 1984; Kroll et al. 1989). In our clinic for Indochinese refugees, PTSD was found to be currently prevalent in 92% of Cambodians, 93% of Mien tribespeople from Laos, and 54% of Vietnamese (Kinzie et al. 1990). Most of the trauma was related to concentration camp experiences, but other traumatic events, including robbery, assault, and rape, also had occurred. Diagnosis was difficult, and often PTSD was found to be present only after a systematic reinterview. Studies in a nonclinical sample of Cambodian adolescents found high rates of depression, and PTSD was present in about 50% of the individuals. However, the depressive symptoms diminished over time, whereas the PTSD symptoms were more persistent and episodic (Kinzie et al. 1986, 1989).

The following case describes a severely traumatized Cambodian refugee, who has been in treatment for 12 years.

Case Report: Phon

Prologue

After the fall of Saigon in 1975, a radical Marxist group in neighboring Cambodia, led by Pol Pot, seized the country and began a reign of terror (Becker 1986). All cities became deserted as the population was rounded up and placed in crude rural work camps, where the ruling regime enforced long labor periods of up to 15 hours without relief and, frequently, a Communist education. Children were separated from their parents, and members of the old regime were singled out for execution. Buddhist monks, merchants, professors, doctors, and military leaders were often subject to brutal, public deaths. Either by design, mismanagement, or creeping paranoia, about one-third of the seven million people in Cambodia died of execution, starvation, or disease. The horror ended in 1979, when Vietnam invaded Cambodia. Phon's story is about one of the survivors.

Clinical Presentation

When first seen, Phon was a 39-year-old Cambodian woman who was referred for evaluation of depression. She gave a history of a very difficult life, aggravated by some current stressors. Her symptoms included nightmares, intrusive thoughts, startle reaction, difficulty falling asleep, poor concentration, and attempts to avoid all memories of the past. Her mood was depressed; she felt guilty and fatigued, and she had lost interest in almost all events in her environment. In the last several months, she had become anorexic, losing 10 pounds. She had suicidal thoughts and had one mild suicide attempt, in which she jumped in front of a moving vehicle. The particular traumas in her life began even before the terrible Pol Pot regime in Cambodia. During her marriage, she had been emotionally and physically abused by her husband. During Pol Pot's time (1975–1979), her mother died of starvation, as did Phon's youngest child. She had thought her husband had died, but later discovered he was alive, although there had been no contact with him and she had thought of herself as widowed. More recently, her children, a daughter and son, who came to the United States with her had become more independent and disrespectful. The daughter had an older boy-friend living in the home, and the patient was upset about this socially embarrassing behavior.

History

Phon was born in a farming community in Cambodia, the eldest of five children. Her father died when she was young. After 3 years of education, she stayed home to take care of her siblings. She had married a farmer who apparently had many affairs and twice left her when she was pregnant, coming back after the second child was born but not returning after the birth of the third child. During the Pol Pot regime, after the death of her youngest child, the patient was separated from her children and, in the 4 years following, was subjected to forced labor. In 1979, she escaped to Thailand and lived there for 5 years, until she came to the United States with her two children. She believed that her siblings were still alive in Cambodia.

Mental Status

On examination, the patient was an attractive looking Cambodian female who appeared slightly older than her stated age and had marked reddening around the eyes. She exhibited psychomotor retardation and appeared very sad. She told her story quite slowly, with little change in expression. There was some crying when she described the past relationship with her husband and the disrespect she felt from her children now. There was no difficulty with cognition, and the affect, although sad, was quite congruent with her stated mood.

Formulation

The patient had multiple traumas in her life, including being the victim of domestic violence, losing a child and a mother to starvation, undergoing 4 years of forced labor and starvation, witnessing brutal acts, and having to escape to Thailand, where she was a refugee for 5 years before coming to the United States. Additionally, she now felt that her children, whom she believed she had saved, were showing "disrespect" for her by their socially inappropriate behavior. At this evaluation, she was diagnosed with PTSD and major depression.

Treatment

The patient was treated over 12 years as part of a program specializing in the treatment of refugees. During this time, the same psychiatrist and Cambodian mental health worker were involved in her case. The program emphasized psychiatric treatment, group therapy, and individual therapy, including help with social and financial problems. These components will be discussed somewhat separately, and then the interventions over the 12 years will be further detailed.

Treatment Components

Early immediate interventions.   At the first session, a stage was set where Phon would feel comfortable and her history could be explored in a straightforward but undemanding way. The patient expressed uncertainty about why she had these symptoms. At the end of the interview, she was given a model that enumerated multiple stressors she had endured over the previous 13 years, which were now causing her symptoms. It was emphasized that she was not becoming crazy, but that even a strong person, such as she, would eventually break down under the tremendous stress, including the final disrespect by her children, which had signified to her that, perhaps, all her efforts to save them had been in vain. She seemed to understand this model. It was further emphasized that she could not commit suicide, because it was her karma to live and care for the children, a fact with which she agreed. She was instructed about the treatment expectations, which included keeping her appointments, not attempting suicide, and taking the medicine as prescribed. Furthermore, a letter was written to a social welfare agency, asking help in obtaining some immediate financial assistance, and she was assisted in filling out the necessary forms.

During the following years, she kept all her appointments, which were weekly for group therapy and about every 6–8 weeks with the psychiatrist for individual therapy. She was prescribed and began taking imipramine for the depression and clonidine for the hyperarousal symptoms and nightmares. This medication changed somewhat over the 12 years, but she continued to take some form of antidepressant medicine.

Group therapy.   Phon joined an ongoing socialization group of other Cambodian refugees, which consisted of 12–15 members led by a Cambodian mental health worker. The intent of the group was to provide a socializing experience in which patients could overcome their own isolation, receive education about living in the United States, and participate in cultural activities and ceremonies. They also began celebrating American holidays, such as Thanksgiving and Christmas. The group encouraged bicultural adaptation, adjusting to living in the United States and maintaining contacts with their own country.

Once a month, for the first 3 years, the group also had the psychiatrist come and do a form of psychotherapy. During this time, there were no activities, just talking and expressing feelings. This process was somewhat complicated, since much of their discussion had to be translated. Nevertheless, the expressed emotion was quite intense, and for the first year the group immediately went back to their experiences during Pol Pot's time and shared their traumas and losses. Recounting and sharing of these experiences, once started, seemed to be unstoppable, and the group therapy became quite intense. After several years, the group was able to discuss other topics, particularly those relating to Cambodia and, eventually, topics pertaining to life in the United States. The most difficult topic pertaining to their present life was raising children in the United States.

It was unclear whether this type of intense expression was helpful; certainly, in the groups it could not be stopped once it had begun. The group members, including Phon, felt it was good to have the doctor there, partly because his presence justified it as a form of treatment. However, there was universal agreement that once a month was enough, since it often took them a week or so to calm down after the intensity of the group therapy.

Individual therapy.   The Cambodian health worker served as interpreter and was with the psychiatrist in the individual sessions, which occurred every 6 weeks to 2 months. At each session, Phon was weighed, had her blood pressure and pulse checked by the nurse, and marked a mood visual analogue scale on a 100-mm line. These measures indicated how the patient was feeling and reacting, physiologically and psychologically. Over time, the therapist acted in several ways: as the physician helping with the symptoms, adjusting and changing medicine as needed; as a trusted advisor on practical matters of living in the United States, PTSD as a reaction to trauma, and the effects of depression; and as an interested listener in the patient's life. Clearly, the subsequent events in Phon's life could not have been predicted, but the ongoing relationship continued with interest, warmth, and a sense of mutual respect.

Major Themes and Progress of Therapy

During the first year, there was a marked reduction in symptoms. Nightmares and reexperiencing of memories were greatly reduced. Phon's sleeping improved, and her depression became less severe. During this year, the patient's blood was tested for imipramine, the level of which proved to be in the therapeutic range. Indeed, she had been compliant with taking her medication.

During the second year, the patient's daughter married, and Phon felt much better about her daughter's more socially appropriate situation. Phon still had had no news from her relatives in Cambodia for over 8 years. She had further reduction in nightmares, but her symptoms increased after she witnessed a car accident and saw the corpse of a friend during a funeral. However, these symptom reactivations were short-lived.

During the third year, her daughter became pregnant, and the prospect of becoming a grandparent pleased Phon. She received some news from Cambodia, and her brother, whom she had not heard from for 9 years, began to ask her for money. This caused much conflict and increased her depressive symptoms. Later, a younger sister also asked for money. Because the patient was quite poor, she felt particularly conflicted. She was given permission in the therapy not to send any more than she could reasonably afford, since taking care of her family here was her primary goal.

During the fourth year, Phon noted that she had a further increase of symptoms while watching violence on television. Other news from Cambodia indicated that her family was doing fine, and a visitor there brought news from her father and siblings. She said that her children were beginning to show her more respect, and she felt more comfortable with them. It is quite likely that the reduction in her symptoms, and perhaps decreased irritability, contributed to this.

In the fifth year, the Gulf War received prominent television attention. Phon showed a marked increase in symptoms and also became very worried about her son's being drafted. She inadvertently went off her medicine for a time, and her symptoms greatly increased. She expressed a sadness about her own life, never having been able to go to school in Cambodia and being unable to work in this country. She became worried about a potential medical problem of a new grandson, but became comforted when testing was done and he was found to be normal.

In the sixth year, Phon's son-in-law brought back a video from Cambodia, and she became quite sad when she saw how poor her sister's family appeared.

During the seventh year, Phon's son-in-law and daughter were having intense domestic problems. She became worried about the grandchildren and about how they were coping with these difficulties. At this time, her son and her daughter's family, including her three grandchildren and her son-in-law, were all living with her. A brother called from Cambodia and said that things were better, although she later heard by letter that there was increased fighting where her family lived, and this caused a marked increase of nightmares and intrusive thoughts. She was able to talk by phone to her father and felt better as a result of this contact.

During the eighth year, Phon said she was much improved, with the exception of having poor concentration and forgetfulness. She was doing well. However, she was not able to cook because she would forget and leave food cooking on the stove, resulting in burnt pots and pans. Periodic talks with her family in Cambodia helped with the general reduction in stress; however, she discovered that her father had become quite ill, and her son-in-law and daughter did not show any "respect" to her. Phon became quite tearful about the conflict with her son-in-law and thought she should move out of her current living situation. During this time, there was a visit with the mental health counselor by the patient and the daughter, at which they were able to work out some of their differences, and Phon felt much improved. This also improved Phon's relationship with her son-in-law, allowing her to stay in her current living situation.

During the tenth year, Phon received news that her estranged husband, who had left her long ago in Cambodia, was, indeed, alive in Cambodia and had taken a second wife and family. She felt very sad about this, and felt quite betrayed, as the second wife was a former friend of hers. She was also ambivalent because her daughter had not yet met her father, and she was unsure whether, in fact, she should. She expressed marked depression and ambivalence, and the memory of her former husband brought back further memories of Cambodia and their complicated and ultimately abusive relationship.

During this time her father was reportedly quite ill and calling out to see Phon before he died. Subsequently, the patient developed marked hypertension, and clonidine, which had been stopped for a time, was restarted. The son-in-law and daughter paid for the patient to return to Cambodia. In Cambodia, she visited her father and sister and felt relieved that they were, in fact, doing moderately well. She felt very conflicted when she saw her former husband. Partly, she was angry about how she had been treated; partly, she was sad that he was so sick and needed the second family to take care of him. She was quite moved when he asked her for forgiveness for the way he had treated her. She returned with a much better affect, reduced depression, and very few symptoms.

During the eleventh year, Phon became concerned and worried about taking the citizenship test. Because of a recent congressional action, she faced the loss of all benefits if she did not become a citizen. This action applied even to refugees with legal status. It helped that an explanation was given, during group therapy, about the necessary procedures for becoming a citizen. At the same time, she found out her father had had a stroke in Cambodia, and she had a marked increase of PTSD symptoms. While studying for the citizenship test, and in part because of her concerns pertaining to the test and her father's health, she again became quite hypertensive. Her first attempt at taking the test was in English, and she failed. She was then given a medical exemption by her psychiatrist to take the test in her native language, which she did, and passed. Getting her citizenship resulted in a reduction in symptoms.

In the twelfth year, she intercepted a call from her ex-husband in Cambodia to her son during which her ex-husband asked for money. She felt very betrayed by his behavior, as she had forgiven him. She also had a conflict with her daughter, because the daughter wanted to sponsor a half sister to come to the United States. This brought back further memories of her abusive husband, but she was able to talk her daughter out of sponsoring the half sister, and she felt much better. During the last part of this year, a very close friend—a young woman with several small children—committed suicide by hanging. For several weeks, Phon had a marked increase in nightmares, which occurred nightly and were associated with much avoidance behavior and fear. She discussed her friend's suicide during therapy sessions, and the nightmares and avoidant behavior diminished. She said at the end of the session, "If I didn't have this clinic and you [meaning the doctor and counselor], I would have committed suicide also."

Interpersonal Aspects of Treatment

The brief patient sketch above only hints at some of the processes involved in the complicated, long-term, cross-cultural interaction called therapy. As the treating psychiatrist for 12 years, I will make personal and subjective comments in addition to the more detached description above. First, this treatment did not occur in isolation. A Cambodian mental health professional and I have had about 80 patients in treatment at any one time in a program that has existed for 20 years. This means we have gained much knowledge about Cambodian refugees, their culture, and their trauma. Through our experiences over the years, our sensitivity, and probably our therapeutic effectiveness, has greatly increased. Second, Phon changed over time, her children grew (one married), she learned some English, and she became a citizen comfortable in American ways—setting up house, shopping, dressing, driving, and interacting with the larger community. Despite this, she remained "Cambodian" in the sense of being shy, respectful, Buddhist, and sensitive to the social perception of her.

Although it may seem a therapeutic leap for a Western-trained psychiatrist to form a long-term relationship with a rural Cambodian refugee, the situation did not feel strained or unique. In our sessions, we developed a shared world. After initial Cambodian greetings, with hands together in front, our conversation had much more to do with the human condition than a specific culture or even the diagnosis. We shared the pains described above, but also the joys—a daughter's marriage, the birth of a grandchild, a son's doing well at school, passing the citizenship test, a father's improving health, and a successful return trip to Cambodia. There was also the fun and humor of sharing the Cambodian celebrations, eating, dancing, taking pictures, and the giving of small gifts that occurred in a group setting.

Beyond all of this was the extreme tragedy of a profoundly traumatized life—4 years of concentration camp experience, with separation from family, forced labor, malnutrition, no medical care, and loss of a mother and a baby to starvation, being surrounded by death and corpses with the possibility of dying herself, and threatened by random killings while trying to escape from Cambodia. These events all resulted from an Indochinese war and the opportunistic takeover of a radical, murderous, Marxist regime. Phon was confronted with these events after she had already endured physical abuse and abandonment by her husband. Her suffering was truly catastrophic, and I have had to restrain my anger that such inhumanity should occur to anyone. There is something terribly wrong with the human condition for people to be able to cause such pain. Along with my anger, there is also the recognition that Phon has somehow survived, admittedly with pain and symptoms, but also with grace and dignity, and without hatred or vindictiveness. This is what her story gives to me and to all of us.

Technical Aspects of Treatment

Although the interpersonal aspects of treatment are probably the most important, there are several technical aspects that deserve mention. First, a large number of patients from Phon's own culture attended the clinic. She, therefore, did not feel alone and isolated. Special ethnic counselors were available, as well as group therapy for members of the same cultural background, and the staff gained knowledge and experience in the culture.

Second, the treatment was long-term and supportive (of a special type) in its approach. There was no indication for brief time-limited therapy, which would tend to minimize the extreme trauma and imply that the disorder could be managed in a short time. Clearly, this was not the case; the trauma and sequelae were profound and enduring, and the patient's life would never be the same as before. Added to the traumatic aspects were the patient's refugee status and her adjustment to a new culture, with different customs, language, economy, government, and complexity. The patient, incidentally, never suggested stopping treatment, and, indeed, she kept all of her appointments for 12 years, indicating her sense of the value of the treatment.

Third, although the therapy was supportive, emphasizing consistency, warm interaction, and dealing with the here and now, psychologically complex issues were often raised. These included a sense of shame about a daughter's living with her boyfriend; conflicts about giving money to relatives in Cambodia, when she had little herself; feelings of being disrespected by her son-in-law; and marked anger and later ambivalence on learning that her former husband had married a good friend. As is typical for many Asians, conflicts often center around complicated family issues, and there may be no culturally safe way to sort out these issues. In this setting, a therapist from another culture can provide a safe, confidential outlet for subjective distress and sometimes help with active approaches to the problems.

Fourth, the therapy was never directed at relieving and/or reframing the severe trauma. Although some therapists working with trauma victims feel the trauma must somehow be worked through, it is doubtful that their patients have had a prolonged death-camp experience, with the catastrophic effects of deaths of relatives, starvation, forced labor, humiliation, and continued threats of death. There is no way to "work though" the trauma. It can be described to, heard, and maybe even understood by the therapist, but it can never be integrated into current life or described in terms of psychological defense mechanisms. It can be remembered as a terrible human tragedy, of which the patient is a survivor who must somehow go on. This approach may aid suppression, or more likely avoidance behavior, and, to the extent that the patient's functioning improves, can be beneficial. Occasionally, patients, after some time in therapy, may want to discuss the trauma, and sessions may be devoted to it. More often, the patients do not refer to it again. However, it is not forgotten, and often, when patients respond to stress in a hyperaroused way or continue to have poor concentration, it is useful to remind them that they have lived with severe stress in the past and that their bodies and minds are still vulnerable to new stress.

Treatment of Traumatized
Southeast Asian Refugees

Cross-cultural psychiatric treatment is difficult, but with traumatized refugees it is even more complex. The patients experience marginalization, minority status, poor physical health, head injuries, collapse of social support, and difficulties adapting to American culture (Ekblad et al. 1998).

The symptoms of PTSD, with nightmares, startle reaction, avoidance behavior, and poor concentration, probably represent a confusing, unique psychological state for which traditional healing does not exist. These factors, adding to the Asian's usual reluctance to seek psychiatric help, mean that patients often wait for treatment for psychological trauma, and when they do receive treatment, it often seems inappropriate to them.

No controlled studies of cross-cultural treatment of traumatized refugees exist. The reports in the literature come from survivors of torture, who often are refugees (Chester and Jaranson 1994). Note that the primary treatment has often been psychotherapy, but no controlled outcome studies have been completed. Others have described treatments that have been useful for victims of torture. These include "insight" therapy (Somnier and Genefke 1986; Vesti and Kastrup 1992), relational therapy (Varvin and Hauff 1998), and short-term treatment for depression and torture survivors (Drees 1989). Cognitive therapy (Basoglu 1992, 1998) and psychodynamic therapy (Allodi 1998; Bustos 1992) have been frequently employed. Other approaches include supportive therapy, desensitization, family groups (Fischman and Ross 1990), and giving testimony (Vesti and Kastrup 1992). Although cognitive therapy has been effective in treating PTSD (Keane et al. 1992), most experienced clinicians feel that severely traumatized individuals require much longer treatment than that offered with the relatively short-term approach of behavior therapy.

The common ingredients of most treatments involve telling the trauma story and then reframing and reworking it (Mollica 1988). Clearly, this process needs to be carried out in a safe setting, with appropriate timing. Even the retelling of the trauma story depends on the patient's cultural experience. For example, South American refugees seem more willing to retell trauma stories and to be helped by the retelling. Indochinese are reluctant to tell about their traumas and often have an exacerbation of symptoms after such therapeutic attempts (Morris and Silove 1992).

Drug therapy has been used for refugee victims of extreme trauma, and Jaranson (1991) stressed the importance of starting medication for highly symptomatic patients, even if evaluation is still in progress. There have been studies to indicate that different doses are needed for non-Caucasians than for Caucasians, and pharmacokinetic (metabolic) and pharmacodynamic (brain receptor) influences have been demonstrated (Lin et al. 1993). The issue is complicated by studies that show very poor compliance among Indochinese patients (Kinzie et al. 1987; Kroll et al. 1989). Among refugees, antidepressants (tricyclics [TCAs] and selective serotonin reuptake inhibitors [SSRIs]) and clonidine have been found useful for some symptoms. The antidepressant effects of TCAs and SSRIs have been used to treat depression and sleep disorder (Kinzie and Edeki 1998). Clonidine has been particularly useful for hyperarousal and nightmare symptoms (Kinzie et al. 1989, 1994).

Most therapies have been useful for reexperiencing hyperarousal symptoms, but rather ineffective for avoidance and numbing symptoms. There is some evidence that long-term socialization group therapy, with an emphasis on a supportive environment, redoing cultural rituals, education about the disorder and medications, and learning to live in an American society, has helped with social isolation and some avoidance behavior (Kinzie et al. 1988).

Treatment Conditions

Phon's treatment illustrates some major points in the therapy of severely traumatized refugee patients. These points must be considered in developing an effective and sensitive treatment program.

1. PTSD in refugees adjusting to new countries is a long-term disability and requires a long-term treatment approach.
2. Treatment needs to be multifaceted and to integrate several interventions: medical, social, group, and individual therapy.
3. The symptoms of PTSD, especially the intrusive symptoms, are very sensitive to stress, and long after periods of remission they can return under stress of any type, such as sight of blood, personal conflicts, reminders of previous trauma, or an intense negative experience.
4. The personal qualities of the psychiatrist and mental health workers are extremely important. A warm, gentle, accepting, genuine, and confidential attitude, which provides consistency and safety, and a free environment in which topics can be discussed are essential.
5. Understanding the patient's culture and history can help the therapist make appropriate interpretations about the patient's feelings and behavior.
6. Existential issues, regarding evil in the universe and the meaning of the suffering of innocent people, are always in the background of the therapy and may promote understanding or severe empathetic strain (see discussion later in this chapter) on the part of the therapist.

Treatment Processes

In providing an optimal program for treatment, there must be a range of services organized with adequate staffing (Kinzie 1991). Within this program, the basis of treatment is the doctor-patient relationship. This relationship depends on the personality and style of the therapist (Kinzie and Fleck 1987). Traumatized refugees are very sensitive to rejection or symbolic threats, and certain personal qualities in the therapist are essential in establishing this relationship. These qualities include genuineness, warmth, empathy, interest in and knowledge about the patient's culture, understanding of the likely traumas the patient faced, and a calmness and acceptance on hearing the trauma story. In short, the therapist needs to like and appreciate the patient. The specific requirements are listed below:

1. *Establish safety.* The patient must be safe, with a guarantee of absolute confidentiality (an important issue with interpreters present) and no pressure to tell or not tell a story.
2. *Promote continuity of care.* It is important that therapists who are taking the history provide an ongoing relationship. There is no place for separation of evaluation and treatment.
3. *Take seriously the patient's symptoms, which are usually somatic, and respect his or her subjective complaints.* Patients rarely come with a trauma story, or even PTSD symptoms, but usually with a variety of somatic complaints, which are often confusing and difficult to integrate.
4. *Take a complete history, including events before and after the trauma.* This helps both therapist and patient put the patient's life in perspective, and provides credibility in the relationship with the patient.
5. *Give an explanatory model appropriate to the patient's culture and symptoms.* The symptoms are often confusing to the patient, and many may even make the patient feel he or she is "going crazy." Most patients are helped by a clear statement that enumerates the stress and the trauma and explains that the mind and body are reacting to these pressures.
6. *Establish a treatment contract and goals.* For refugees who are depressed and have low self-esteem, negotiations with an American professional may not be easy or even completely appropriate. A useful approach is to state the likely early goals—improved sleep, improved mood, and a reduction in nightmares—and ask if there are other aspects that need to be worked on.
7. *Provide relief of symptoms.* In the first session, it is usually necessary to start medication to provide relief, even if the evaluation is not complete. Medicine not only provides help with distressing symptoms but also often fits with the role of the Western physician and provides a sense of the therapist's competency to treat the patient's needs. This treatment is often not difficult, because a variety of medicines are effective.

8. *Provide environmental safety.* Refugees face multiple ongoing problems, and an effective clinic needs to address these problems through the physician and case managers. Their role includes contacting social agencies regarding welfare income, housing, and medical assistance.

9. *Provide continuity of therapeutic themes.* In ongoing contact, the patient and therapist develop a steady, safe relationship—one based on issues and themes. Often, these themes continue around losses from the previous country, such as death of family, loss of social relationships, and, frequently, financial losses. In addition, there are ongoing problems of adjusting to a new country and dealing with unfamiliar laws and customs, and more disturbing issues of raising children with problems such as drugs and gangs. For some, a therapist listens and supports, and for others, he or she offers practical advice, suggestions, and information about living in the new country.

10. *Give the patient freedom to tell the trauma story in his or her own way.* How to handle the trauma story is a difficult clinical decision. Patients often tell their stories in an incomplete, disconnected, and emotionally packed manner. They often feel relieved and unburdened by telling their stories and by having been listened to and understood. However, many will find that the interview will stimulate memories and that there may be an exacerbation of nightmares and intrusive thoughts for a time. Some ethnic groups will gain intellectual mastery and integration in their lives, through exploration of internal problems associated with torture at the hands of political opponents. Others find acceptance and avoidance as the most adaptive approach. The best clinical strategy is to follow the patient's lead in approaching or avoiding extensive trauma discussion. However, when the patient has marked nightmares and hyperarousal symptoms, further stimulation may need to be postponed for a time.

The most important aspect is to clearly recognize that the effects of massive trauma, deaths, torture, concentration camps, and loss of country can never be fully understood or integrated. Life will never be the same. The losses are real are permanent, and they bring into question the meaning of life, pain, and even death. There is no quick fix, and a promise of rapid cure will ring false and shallow. Sometimes, the authentic position is to stay and be with the patient through the pain. The sharing of the experience decreases isolation and brings two people of markedly different backgrounds and experiences closer. There may be no better therapy than this.

Countertransference and Empathetic Strain

Treating trauma patients is exceedingly difficult. The therapist must confront pain and suffering but also sustain empathy. However, as treatment unfolds, it may be increasingly difficult to stay tuned in to the patient because of transference feelings, which result in *empathetic strain*. As Wilson and Lindy (1994) point out, empathetic strain can result in two different reactions. One involves avoidance, distancing, and detachment, and the other involves overidentification, enmeshment, and excessive advocacy. In studies with our staff in the Indochinese Psychiatric Program, we found that counselors differed significantly from the psychiatrists in their reactions (Kinzie 1994). In our survey of the reactions, the six counselors from Southeast Asia (two Vietnamese, two Laotian, and two Cambodian) all denied any problems of personal reactions, including avoidance behavior, irritability, or even sadness, at hearing the stories. However, among the counselors, we observed frequent avoidance of patients, anger at some patients, and at times much limiting of their contact with patients. They tended to exhibit detachment and distancing behavior.

On the other hand, the four psychiatrists, including myself, readily recognized a wide variety of complex responses. These included, during the patient's sessions, a general sense of sadness; anger, irritability, and hyperarousal; and excessive identification with the patients. These responses were often felt as sadness over the patient's tragedy, anger with the perpetrators of the violence, and a sense of being uniquely able to protect the patient from further trauma. In addition, we all felt that we developed an intolerance to the conflicts and losses of others (nonrefugees). It is difficult to be sensitive to the needs of someone who has lost a job, failed a college course, or been separated from a spouse, after interviewing a patient who describes her husband and children being killed and has endured years of forced labor and starvation.

Although not technically countertransference, a series of reactions occurred among the psychiatrists. Most of us noticed an increasing intolerance of violence—the abhorrence of watching violence on television and films, or even disgust at news reports of fights, rapes, and murder. (In my own case, I have not watched war movies, especially about Vietnam or Cambodia, for 20 years.) There was also a personal sense of vulnerability. Knowing that savage brutality can occur in a quiet Buddhist country like Cambodia means it can occur anyplace (a fact underlined by the nightly news), and we are all vulnerable to unspeakable and unpredictable horrors. There is another sense of living a personal myth. "I know the evil that occurs in other people and

I (only I?) can help." The myth can take on tragic dimensions, such as the unending burden of Sisyphus, or heroic dimensions, such as the protection of helpless people by the Seven Samurai.

Beyond the personal reactions, there was a broader reaction of a sense of the failure of Western medicine and psychiatry. Nothing in my medical or psychiatric education prepared me or even warned me that I would be treating patients whose disorders were caused by evil done by others. Did none of my teachers know about this? Perhaps the failure was even beyond education. The Enlightenment, with its optimism about human discovery, permeated Western and American culture, yet those immersed in that culture did not seem to be able to confront or even recognize the inhumanity in how people treat each other. Is there some fatal flaw in humans that our culture and society do not admit to or understand? Is there something terribly wrong with our understanding of human nature? Such doubts linger long after the patient leaves, and even after the patient improves.

There are ways that will enhance a clinician's ability to cope with the effects of treating massively traumatized patients:

• Working on normal therapeutic issues, which often are the major part of therapy
• Obtaining satisfaction with the patient's improvement
• Maintaining scientific and professional curiosity about trauma and PTSD
• Limiting the number of traumatized patients one treats

Above all, a sense of support of and respect for colleagues at a personal and professional level maintains objectivity and reduces the effects of isolation.

Conclusion

The treatment of refugees from Southeast Asia is difficult, since differences in language, culture, and expectations of treatment between the psychiatrist and patient may be quite marked. The experience of massive psychological trauma, with total disruption of an individual's life and sense of security and the addition of depressive and PTSD symptoms, makes treatment even more difficult. Cultural and personal identities influence how trauma is handled, but to a substantial degree many victims develop similar symptoms and behaviors that persist for a long time and have a marked tendency to recur. The treatment needs to work with both the patient's culture and his or her personal trauma experience. The major therapeutic ingredients provide safety, support, consistency, a long-term doctor-patient relationship, and mutually acceptable goals. Therapy also needs to address the multiple themes that surface in the therapeutic work, provide symptomatic relief with medication, and carefully and sensitively work with the trauma story, especially when symptoms recur. Helping traumatized refugees involves high demands on the therapist, but the rewards can be very satisfying.

References

Allodi F: The physician's role in assessing and treating torture and the PTSD syndrome, in Caring for Victims of Torture. Edited by Jaranson J, Popkin M. Washington, DC, American Psychiatric Press, 1998, pp 89–106

American Psychiatric Association: Diagnostic and Statistical Manual of Mental Disorders, 3rd Edition. Washington, DC, American Psychiatric Association, 1980

Basoglu M: Behavioural and cognitive approach in the treatment of torture-related psychological problems, in Torture and Its Consequences: Current Treatment Approaches. Edited by Basoglu M. Cambridge, UK, Cambridge University Press, 1992, pp 402–429

Basoglu M: Behavioral and cognitive treatment of survivors of torture, in Caring for Victims of Torture. Edited by Jaranson J, Popkin M. Washington, DC, American Psychiatric Press, 1998, pp 131–148

Becker E: When the War Was Over: The Voices of Cambodia's Revolution and Its People. New York, Simon & Schuster, 1986

Boehnlein JK, Kinzie JD, Rath B, et al: One year follow-up study of post-traumatic stress disorder among survivors of Cambodian concentration camps. Am J Psychiatry 142:956–959, 1985

Bustos E: Psychodynamic approaches in the treatment of torture survivors, in Torture and Its Consequences: Current Treatment Approaches. Edited by Basoglu M. Cambridge, UK, Cambridge University Press, 1992, pp 333–347

Chester B, Jaranson J: The context of survival and destruction: conducting psychotherapy with survivors of torture. National Center for Post Traumatic Stress Disorder Clinical Newsletter 4:17–20, 1994

Drees A: Guidelines for a short-term therapy of a torture depression. J Trauma Stress 2:549–554, 1989

Ekblad S, Kohn R, Jansson B: Psychological and cultural aspects of immigration and mental health, in Clinical Methods in Transcultural Psychiatry. Edited by Okpaku SO. Washington, DC, American Psychiatric Press, 1998, pp 42–66

Fischman Y, Ross J: Group treatment of exiled survivors of torture. Am J Orthopsychiatry 60:135–142, 1990

Jaranson J: Psychotherapeutic medication, in Mental Health Services for Refugees (DHHS Publ No ADM-91-1824). Edited by Westermeyer J, Williams CL, Nguyen AN. Washington, DC, U.S. Government Printing Office, 1991, pp 132–145

Keane TM, Albano AM, Blake DD: Current trends in the treatment of post-traumatic stress symptoms, in Torture and Its Consequences: Current Treatment Approaches. Edited by Basoglu M. Cambridge, UK, Cambridge University Press, 1992, pp 363–401

Kinzie JD: Development, staffing and structure of psychiatric clinics, in Mental Health Services for Refugees (DHHS Publ No ADM-91-1824). Edited by Westermeyer J, Williams CL, Nguyen AN. Washington, DC, U.S. Government Printing Office, 1991, pp 146–156

Kinzie JD: Countertransference in the treatment of Southeast Asian refugees, in Countertransference in the Treatment of PTSD. Edited by Wilson JP, Lindy JD. New York, Guilford, 1994, pp 249–262

Kinzie JD, Edeki T: Ethnicity and psychopharmacology: the experience of Southeast Asians, in Clinical Methods in Transcultural Psychiatry. Edited by Okpaku SO. Washington, DC, American Psychiatric Press, 1998, pp 171–190

Kinzie JD, Fleck J: Psychotherapy with severely traumatized refugees. Am J Psychother 41:82–94, 1987

Kinzie JD, Manson SM: Five-years' experience with Indochinese refugee patients. Journal of Operational Psychiatry 14:105–111, 1983

Kinzie JD, Fredrickson RH, Rath B, et al: Post-traumatic stress disorder among survivors of Cambodian concentration camps. Am J Psychiatry 141:645–650, 1984

Kinzie JD, Sack WH, Angell RH, et al: The psychiatric effects of massive trauma on Cambodian children, I: the children. Journal of the American Academy of Child Psychiatry 25:370–376, 1986

Kinzie JD, Leung P, Boehnlein J, et al: Antidepressant blood levels in Southeast Asians: clinical and cultural implications. J Nerv Ment Dis 175:480–485, 1987

Kinzie JD, Leung P, Bui A, et al: Cultural factors in group therapy with Southeast Asian refugees. Community Ment Health J 24:157–166, 1988

Kinzie JD, Sack WH, Angell RH, et al: A three-year follow-up of Cambodian young people traumatized as children. Journal of the American Academy of Child Psychiatry 28:501–504, 1989

Kinzie J, Boehnlein J, Leung P, et al: The prevalence of posttraumatic stress disorder and its clinical significance among Southeast Asian refugees. Am J Psychiatry 147:913–917, 1990

Kinzie JD, Sack RL, Riley CM: The polysomnographic effects of clonidine on sleep disorders in posttraumatic stress disorder: a pilot study with Cambodian patients. J Nerv Ment Dis 182:585–587, 1994

Kroll J, Habenicht M, Mackenzie T, et al: Depression and posttraumatic stress disorder in Southeast Asian refugees. Am J Psychiatry 146:1592–1597, 1989

Lin K, Poland R, Nagasaki G (eds): Psychopharmacology and Psychobiology of Ethnicity. Washington, DC, American Psychiatric Press, 1993

Mollica R: The trauma story: the psychiatric care of refugee survivors of violence and torture, in Post-traumatic Therapy and Victims of Violence. Edited by Ochberg FM. New York, Brunner/Mazel, 1988, pp 295–314

Mollica R: Southeastern Asian refugees: migration, history and mental health issues, in Amidst Peril and Pain: The Mental Health and Well-Being of the World's Refugees. Edited by Marsella A, Bornemann J, Ekblad S, et al. Washington, DC, American Psychological Association, 1994, pp 83–100

Morris P, Silove D: Cultural influences in psychotherapy with refugee survivors of torture and trauma. Hospital and Community Psychiatry 43:820–824, 1992

Somnier FE, Genefke IK: Psychotherapy for victims of torture. Br J Psychiatry 149: 323–329, 1986

Varvin S, Hauff E: Psychotherapy with patients who have been tortured, in Caring for Victims of Torture. Edited by Jaranson J, Popkin M. Washington, DC, American Psychiatric Press, 1998, pp 117–130

Vesti P, Kastrup K: Psychotherapy for torture survivors, in Torture and Its Consequences: Current Treatment Approaches. Edited by Basoglu M. Cambridge, UK, Cambridge University Press, 1992, pp 348–362

Wilson JP, Lindy JD (eds): Countertransference in the Treatment of PTSD. New York, Guilford, 1994

CHAPTER 13

The Adolescent

Danilo E. Ponce, M.D.

This chapter intends to sort out the complexities inherent in discussing cultural considerations in psychotherapy of the adolescent. An attempt is made to identify the important things that a psychotherapist from one culture ought to know if he or she is to be reasonably successful in treating an adolescent from another culture.

At the outset, it might be useful to point out Vargas and Koss-Chioino's (1992) cogent observation that describing effective cross-cultural psychotherapeutic work with adolescents as "culture-sensitive," "culture-relevant," or "culture-informed"—terms that are widely used and favored in academic circles—does *not* really capture the desired process involved. These phrases convey, perhaps unintentionally, a kind of detached passivity, as if to be "aware," to be "knowledgeable," or to be "pertinent" is enough to guarantee some degree of success in cross-cultural work with adolescents. Vargas and Koss-Chioino contend that this is not enough and that if the clinician is to have any reasonable hope in succeeding in cross-cultural therapy with adolescents, he or she has to be able to transform these "sensitivities" and "sensibilities" into *interactive* or *participatory* competencies—that is, a complex of requisite knowledge, attitudes, skills, and experiences. Hence, Vargas and

Koss-Chioino recommend using the phrase (which we will be using in the rest of this chapter) "culture-responsive" instead.

It also needs to be pointed out that adolescents, cultures, and psycho-therapeutic practices are currently in a state of great flux, especially in the United States, such that to speak of these subjects in a vacuum, as if they are quasi-permanent entities from which timeless verities may be stated, may be not only misleading but disingenuous. Any discussion of these subjects, therefore, will have to mention, in context, qualifiers or caveats regarding contemporary developments that may be impinging on them and, in some important ways, significantly altering their very nature. A timely example is the profound impact of the managed care system in the United Sates (Geraty et al. 1992) in significantly dictating, in just a few short years, what psycho-therapeutic services are provided, how these services are defined, who is providing these services, and how long these services are to be provided. Along the same line, rapid technological advances that are literally quite breathtaking have managed to make the world not only a "global village" (McLuhan 1968; see also Iyer 1993) but, more accurately, an "information autobahn."

Because of these and other facts of contemporary life, the nature of ad-olescence, families, culture, and psychotherapeutic practices is changing drastically. For example, when we refer to "family" now (at least in the Unit-ed States), more often than not it denotes a single parent (usually a mother) with children, and other increasingly frequent permutations, such as homo-sexual couples raising children. Gone is the traditional notion of family as a "nuclear family," consisting of a mother, a father, and children plus an "ex-tended family" of grandparents, aunts, and uncles. With the dissolution and/or fragmentation of the family as we know it, there is a corresponding ripple effect on adolescence and adolescents. Taffel (1996), for instance, describes the notion of a "second family" (e.g., peer groups, youth gangs) now being more significantly influential in a contemporary adolescent's life than the "first family" (i.e., parents).

It does not take a huge amount of wisdom or ingenuity to figure out that technological advances are eroding traditional cultures as we know them, substituting values and belief systems grossly or subtly put out by television networks such as MTV (Music Television) and CNN (Cable Network News) and shows such as *Baywatch* (a program very popular with adolescents, con-sisting mostly of young males and females in various stages of undress). Such erosion of traditional values and beliefs is being experienced by adoles-cents not just in the United States but worldwide—thanks to a global net-work of instant information services (e.g., Internet, satellite television, fax, pagers, e-mail, videophones), in addition to the "old" modes of information dissemination, such as books, magazines, newspapers, radio, and broadcast television.

With these preliminary caveats in mind, it is fair to say that there are still some fundamental, and some not so fundamental, competencies that a psychotherapist desiring to work with adolescents in a cross-cultural situation ought to acquire. We will now examine these competencies.

Cultural Perspectives on Adolescent Development

When doing psychotherapy with adolescents, it is most important to remember that they undergo three distinct developmental substages (Shafer and Irwin 1991): early adolescence (ages 10–13 years); middle adolescence (ages 14–16 years), and late adolescence (ages 17–21 years). Each of these substages has issues that are substantially different from those of the other two and that significantly influence the expression of psychopathology and how it is dealt with in psychotherapy.

In *early adolescence,* issues are primarily organized around puberty and hormonal changes and on the corresponding impact of these changes on the youngster and the systems surrounding him or her. One may say that at this substage the youngster is saddled with the task of mastering same-sex issues (e.g., initiation into youth gangs or cliques). In *middle adolescence,* on the other hand, the youngster, with some life experiences now under his or her belt in dealing with same-sex issues, is poised to explore opposite-sex issues. Hence, tasks and activities are more or less bisexual, having a "push-pull" quality of wanting to be with one's same-sex friends, while being drawn to the "significant other." The security of the gang is slowly shared with the excitement of a dyadic partnership—the youngster "falls in love." In *late adolescence,* the youngster, emerging from the struggles of the previous two substages, is more focused on gearing up for the final goodbye to childhood and formal initiation into the world of grown-ups.

Culture impacts these three adolescent substages by 1) *shaping* acceptable responses, or ways of dealing with substage issues; 2) *legitimizing* responses that are socially acceptable, even if these responses may be at variance with those of the adolescent's peers; 3) *providing rules and injunctions* ("do's" and "don'ts") designed to maintain the acceptable responses (i.e., "reward" compliance and "punish" noncompliance); and 4) *modeling* how these acceptable responses are practiced in day-to-day life.

An example of the impact of culture on adolescent developmental substages is how the issues of sex, sexuality, and gender-identity formation (masculinity and femininity) are handled very differently by various cultures during the adolescent period. In Chinese culture (Char et ål. 1980), there is a pervading atmosphere of sexual neutrality; hence, masculinity, femininity, sex, and sexuality are not issues that are discussed and/or handled freely or openly in the family. One may surmise, therefore, that for the early- and middle-adolescent Chinese youngster, these issues are dealt with mainly through discrete, nonverbal means, such as role modeling by parents and close family members, and tacit and implicit injunctions that the youngster learns through trial and error. The implication for psychotherapy seems clear: bringing up these issues too prematurely or abruptly with a Chinese adolescent (especially in the earlier developmental substages) may put an unnecessary burden on the therapeutic process, risking abrupt termination of the therapeutic alliance.

In contrast, the Filipino culture is decidedly patriarchal and male (*machismo*) oriented, and attitudes toward gender identity, sex, and sexuality revolve around the so-called double standard, by which females are expected to be pure and chaste, while males are encouraged to have "many conquests" (Ponce 1986). From early adolescence onward, the subtle and sometimes not-so-subtle message to the Filipino male is for him to be a "lady killer," and to the female, to be a "Madonna" (the "Virgin Mother" kind, not the entertainer). Psychotherapy with the Filipino early-adolescent male must, therefore, be sensitive to the cultural pressures put upon him to be tough (*macho*) or at least to have a tough exterior. As he progresses to middle adolescence, he is expected to add to this tough exterior numerous amorous conquests. The Filipino president, Joseph Estrada, epitomized this Filipino male ideal in numerous B-movie roles, in which he portrayed rugged characters with guns ablazing and numerous ladies swooning at his feet.

Given the differences and nuances inherent in the adolescent substages and the impact culture has on them, psychotherapeutic interventions must be tailored to fit the developmental substage, taking into account the overarching cultural context. This is of particular importance in dealing with the suicidal adolescent (Potter et al. 1998). To an early adolescent, for example, a suicidal threat or attempt could be a reaction to being excluded from "the group."

The Early Adolescent: The Case of Laura

Laura, age 11, was a recently arrived immigrant from the Philippines who was referred by her school counselor for mental health services because "she looked depressed, and her teachers said she was talking about running away from home, and killing herself." Upon examination, Laura mentioned that her peers in school teased her about the way she spoke and her "funny clothes." They would not let her join them in any extracurricular activities. She said she "didn't have anybody to talk to," because her parents were busy working; an older sister, age 16, was "with her boyfriend all the time"; and her 13-year-old brother was "with his gang."

A Filipino female social worker was assigned to Laura for school-based individual psychotherapy. The therapeutic strategy was to have Laura join a choir in a church group near her home, and psychotherapy emphasized the need for her to be a "good girl," and not to be a problem to her parents, who were "busy making your family's life better." She was seen six times on a weekly basis and then on a monthly basis after that. She reported being happy with her friends in the choir, she was getting good grades in school, and, following the advice of her friends in the choir, she began to dress and behave more appropriately.

Discussion

The strategy adopted reflected consideration of Laura's developmental substage, and a culturally responsive intervention was designed that was sensitive to the Filipino cultural mandate for her to be a "good girl." Another consideration was the need for psychotherapy in early adolescence to be less talk and more action-oriented—hence, the strategy of getting her to join a church choir near her home.

A middle adolescent, on the other hand, may view suicide as providing some sort of relief from the pain of a broken love affair or a messy love triangle. As mentioned earlier, culture plays a role in providing the injunctions and in shaping the responses (e.g., suicide) that are acceptable once injunctions are deemed to have been violated.

The Middle Adolescent: The Case of Tran

Tran, age 14, a girl of Vietnamese ancestry, was taken to the emergency room of a local hospital by her sister Wen, age 16, and her sister's boyfriend, following Tran's ingestion of "about 16 Tylenol pills," ostensibly in an attempt to kill herself. Apparently, her sister's boyfriend had secretly also been seeing Tran. When her sister found out, Tran swallowed the pills because she had "betrayed" her sister and "brought shame to the family."

Tran received follow-up care in individual psychotherapy at an outpatient clinic. The issue of shame became central in therapy, and eventually Tran's sister and parents were brought in to bring closure to the issue (Tran's sister broke off with her boyfriend shortly after the incident). It was clarified by the therapist that although Tran must take responsibility for allowing herself to get involved with her sister's boyfriend, her sister and the ex-boyfriend must also take proportionate responsibility for the respective parts they played—the ex-boyfriend for knowingly and maliciously pursuing her while still attached to her sister, and her sister for not keeping a watchful eye on her boyfriend. The message was that there were no "innocent victims." The parents followed the therapist's lead in spreading the blame, and there was a tearful and emotionally touching reconciliation between Tran and her sister.

Discussion

Significant others, and how to relate to them, become important in middle adolescence. In Tran's case, the cultural values of "shame" and "respect for elders" immediately put the onus of blame on her, and in her mind the only acceptable way to rectify the situation was to kill herself. The therapist, capitalizing on his leverage as an "elder" and an "authority," reconfigured the situation by "spreading blame all around." This allowed Tran to "save face" and enabled Tran and her sister to forgive each other.

A late adolescent contemplates suicide more or less as a solution to a perception that he or she has failed his or her initiation into the grown-up world. In this instance, culture significantly influences the definition of "failure" (or "success," for that matter) and the acceptable responses for having failed (e.g., suicide).

The Late Adolescent: The Case of Tony

Tony, age 19, of Chinese ancestry, was an out-of-state college student. His mother was a well-known physician in her community, respected for her humanitarian and charitable work. His father was a prosperous businessman. Tony was the youngest and the only male of three children. His mother got a frantic call one day from a distant relative residing near her son's school, saying that Tony had not been attending school, was not taking care of himself, and had muttered something about "disappearing from this world" and "life not worth living anymore." His mother persuaded a psychiatrist colleague to talk to Tony over the phone. Tony revealed to the psychiatrist that he felt he had failed his parents and let them down, because they so desperately wanted him to be a doctor, and he wanted, in his "heart of hearts," to be a chef instead. He thought that by killing himself, he would spare his parents disappointment and grief.

His father took Tony home and arrangements were made for him to see the psychiatrist. He agreed to take antidepressant medications and to come for psychotherapy twice a week. In therapy, he reiterated his overwhelming sense of guilt and shame for not living up to his parent's expectations, but he mentioned quite despondently that he could no longer "live a life of lies." A family therapy session was arranged including both parents, and in that session Tony learned, quite ironically, that his father was a "frustrated Chinese chef." His mother also told him that although she would be quite happy "if he decided to be a doctor," she really would not be disappointed if he decided on some other career. There was a lot of crying in the session by all three. In the next few sessions, Tony decided to go back to college, with the proviso that he would "keep an open mind," and in the meantime he would take some night classes in Chinese cooking in a nearby community college.

Discussion

Tony's struggles are characteristic of the late adolescent's lament, "Who am I going to be?" Conflicts are usually defined in terms of who the adolescent thinks he *ought* to be versus who he *wants* to be. In traditional cultures, the former almost always wins out in the end. With modernization, cultural supports are eroding, such that the balance is shifting in the direction of "want to be" for the late adolescent. In Tony's case, his dilemma was helped immensely by the family therapy session, which clarified his misperception of the "ought to be's."

Clinical Worldviews of the Psychotherapist Working With Adolescents

Most, if not all, the research studies on the efficacy of psychotherapy (albeit mostly with the adult population) have shown that it is the psychotherapist's *personality*, as well as his or her ability to instill hope and overcome demoralization, that seems to be the one constant variable in determining psychotherapeutic success or failure (Bergin 1971; Frank 1991; Russell 1994). The psychotherapist's personality becomes doubly important in providing culturally responsive therapy to adolescents for reasons that will be discussed in more detail later. For now, in the context of talking about psychotherapy, "personality" is probably best understood in terms of the psychotherapist's *clinical worldviews*. Clinical worldviews, or what Frank (1991) calls "assumptive worlds," are the therapist's core beliefs or values regarding diagnoses (i.e., nature of health, disease, or illness), treatment (i.e., therapy, cure, or management of the diagnoses), and prognosis (i.e., predicted outcome, with or without treatment). It is these internal, and usually implicit, belief systems that the psychotherapist relies on to collect information, exclude information, formulate a hypothesis, and implement interventions.

Examples of these clinical worldview models are the *biological* (i.e., neurological, genetic, neurochemical), *psychological* (i.e., affective, behavioral, cognitive), and *social* (i.e., group, family, social class). If the psychotherapist's clinical worldview is predominantly psychological—and more specifically, cognitive-behavioral—it is of course not surprising that the therapist will be looking for "irrational ideas that lead to stupid behaviors" as a diagnostic consideration and using "vigorous challenging of these irrational ideas" as a treatment prescription. The same process holds true when one is attached to biological or social clinical worldviews.

Cultural factors impact the psychotherapist by 1) *shaping* or heavily influencing the psychotherapist's clinical worldviews; 2) *dictating* what issues are legitimately dealt with in the therapy (e.g., transference and countertransference issues dealing with aggression, sex, sexuality, gender identity, power struggles) and therapeutic taboos; 3) *determining* the nature of the interventions and the form the interventions will take (e.g., "Should I deal with the youngster alone in individual therapy, or see the family too?"); and 4) *framing* how therapeutic "success" or "failure" outcomes will be defined and measured.

More often than not, the effects of cultural conditioning on the psychotherapist, though ubiquitous, are subtle and often unrecognized, and therefore deadly when one works with adolescents. As alluded to earlier, the therapist's "personality" (i.e., clinical worldviews conditioned by cultural factors) becomes doubly important in determining therapeutic outcome in working with adolescents, because they, as a rule, 1) have not yet mastered the art of "political correctness"; 2) have not adequately established defense and coping mechanisms, particularly with regard to sexual and aggressive impulses; and 3) are very sensitive to "identity" issues and to feeling "understood." Hence, adolescents tend to act on their feelings and impulses. They generally vote with their feet in therapy and are quite unforgiving ("no second chance") with therapists whom, rightly or wrongly, they perceive as insensitive, who do not "understand" them, and who do not validate or recognize their cultural values.

These considerations are quite important, for example, in therapeutic issues regarding *independence* and *autonomy*. Raised in a culture steeped in valuing independence and self-sufficiency, Western psychotherapists will undoubtedly be guided by these values in their therapeutic work with adolescents and their families. In other cultures, however, most notably in Asian cultures, the preferred movement is centripetal rather than centrifugal: a son is a son, and a daughter is a daughter, for the rest of their lives. Therapeutic impasses usually occur when this particular issue is not recognized by the therapist. This point will be illustrated by the following case example:

> Dr. Smith, a 29-year-old Caucasian male, is a child and adolescent psychiatry resident from Texas. His patient, Jimmy, is a 17-year-old Vietnamese of Chinese ancestry. In this particular therapy session, Dr. Smith was exhorting the youngster to be more assertive toward his parents, as part of an overall treatment goal of enhancing his "independent living skills."

> **Dr. Smith:** You need to speak up more to your parents, Jimmy. I'd like you to tell them how angry you are when they continue to treat you like a child.
> **Jimmy:** I don't know . . . I can't do that.
> **Dr. Smith:** What do you mean you can't do that? You'll be an adult in a few months. What's the matter, you scared of them or something?
> **Jimmy:** No. It's just that we don't do those kinds of things in my family.
> **Dr. Smith:** Well. You just gotta do it.

One other issue pertaining to the psychotherapist that deserves special attention is that of countertransference, especially countertransference surrounding erotic reactions generated in the therapy session. It is axiomatic that in conducting therapy with adolescents, it is not a matter of "if," but "when" and "how" erotic countertransference reactions are to be handled (Ponce 1993). Culture complicates the picture, because, as previously mentioned, various cultures have different ways of dealing with gender identity, sex, and sexuality. It is beyond the scope of this chapter to discuss further how the therapist might deal with erotic countertransference reactions (for a more detailed treatment, see Ponce 1993), but suffice it to say that psychotherapists doing cross-cultural work with adolescents will need to be aware of whatever unresolved issues they might have regarding their own sexuality and take the appropriate steps to limit the presence of these issues in the therapeutic process. Otherwise, the potential for acting out countertransference reactions in the therapeutic situation is enormous. This is especially of concern in cross-cultural therapy work with adolescents, in which the countertransference reaction of "exotic is erotic" is quite common. This issue is illustrated by the following case example:

> Dr. Jones, a 28-year-old Caucasian psychologist, worked for a residential treatment program and was the psychotherapist of Malia, a 17-year-old

part-Hawaiian girl. In the course of therapy, Malia managed to make Dr. Jones feel "unique" and "special" and that "only" he could solve her problems (drug use, family problems, some prostitution to support her drug use). When she was discharged from the program upon turning 18, Dr. Jones resigned from the program, continued to see Malia, and married her a year later.

Specific Psychotherapeutic Considerations

Independence Versus Dependence

The adolescent is in the interesting "neither fish nor fowl" status of not being a child anymore by virtue of the simple expedient that with puberty, he or she can now be a father or mother, and yet not being an adult in terms of social and legal rights and privileges. This Janus-like situation creates some interesting paradoxes and dilemmas in therapy. For example, adolescents' dependent status makes the therapeutic contract with them similar to one with children, involving sanction, consent, and/or authorization by a third party, usually the parents or legal custodians (although the age at consent has steadily gone down; in most of the United States, it is now 14 years). At the same time, they are expected to act like adults, behave independently, and be held accountable for their actions. This "damned if you do, damned if you don't" situation is typical of adolescent life and probably accounts for much of the stereotypical *sturm und drang* ("storm and stress") characterization of the adolescent that, despite the heroic efforts of Daniel Offer and associates (Offer and Schonert-Reichl 1992) to scientifically disprove, somehow manages to survive and prosper.

The independence versus dependence issue is peculiar only in cultures where adolescence as a psychosociocultural status exists, such as North American and European cultures. In other cultures or countries where there is an urgent need for another "extra hand" to support the family economically, adolescence as a social status simply does not exist; there is only being a "child" and being an "adult" (Ariès 1961; Demos and Demos 1969). The implication is obvious: therapeutic issues of dependence versus independence—in fact, the whole notion of psychotherapy with adolescents—are relevant only in cultures where adolescence is clearly established as a distinct psychosociocultural state.

The issue of independence versus dependence also can become important with families who migrated from another culture. There is usually a wide value gap between parents and their adolescent children on this issue, often creating conflict between generations. The parents are usually conservative, expecting close, interdependent family relationships. On the other hand, the adolescent is likely to be more acculturated to the host society that encourages independence. This can be a great challenge for the therapist, requiring sensitivity and reflection on his or her own values.

Involvement of Parents in Therapy

Recalling our previous discussion on clinical worldviews, if the therapist subscribes to the view that psychopathology exists in *individuals* (the so-called medical model), it logically follows that attempts to correct the psychopathology will involve interventions targeting the adolescent (e.g., psychotropic medications, individual psychotherapy). If the therapist adheres to the view that psychopathology exists in *relationships between individuals* (the so-called systems model), treatment attempts not only will include the family but will often think of the family as "the patient." The thrust of a third view fixes the psychopathology in the adolescent but actively solicits the help of the family in achieving the therapeutic goals (the so-called middle of the road or eclectic model, i.e., seeing the youngster in individual therapy or giving him or her medications, while involving the parents in "parent education").

There is no inherently right or wrong approach in terms of whether or not to involve the parents or family in therapy, and the decision is likely to depend on the therapist's clinical worldview. Cultural considerations become important when there is an unrecognized and unacknowledged clash of cultural views regarding parental or family involvement in therapy. For instance, in most Asian or patriarchal cultures, the prevalent view is that psychopathology exists in individuals. The message is thus "fix my son/daughter," and any attempts to involve parents or family other than as sources of relevant information and history will usually be met with puzzlement, if not outright resistance and hostility.

How can therapeutic problems surrounding this issue be prevented? First, the therapist can include the parents' and family's worldview(s) of psychopathology, treatment, and ideal treatment outcomes as part of the overall assessment. Second, on the basis of everybody's (adolescent's, parents', other family members', and, of course, therapist's) worldviews, the therapist then designs strategies to fit and/or match.

With Asian parents, for example, it may be more useful to invite the parents' participation in therapy—not to "treat" them, but to involve them in helping their adolescent. The parents are not identified as the source of the adolescent's problems, but as the sources of power who can influence their offspring to improve. This framework or approach will help the parents to save face and, at the same time, maximize the potential impact of the parents in resolving the problems that exist within the family.

Cultural Gap Between Adolescent and Parents

There is a built-in cultural gap between adolescents and their parents that is better known as a "generation gap." As with the weather, there is much talk about this gap but very little that is done about it in a therapy context. A model that might be clinically useful in cross-cultural psychotherapeutic work between adolescents and their parents is Kluckhohn and Strodtbeck's (1961) *value-orientation model*.

According to Kluckhohn and Strodtbeck, there are five "common human problems" and three "fundamental ways of solving these problems." These problems and solutions are seen in terms of how people deal with time (past, present, future); activity (being, being-in-becoming, doing); relation to others (hierarchical, democratic, individualistic); relation to nature/supernature (subjugation, harmony, mastery); and innate human nature (evil, neutral, fixed). An individual's value-orientation profile can be ascertained from a survey form designed to elicit his or her preferred responses to the five "common human problems." The busy clinician, can, of course, use the dimensions as guidelines, relying on the old standby, clinical observations, to see if patterns emerge on the five dimensions. The therapist does not have to cover all five dimensions. Usually, it becomes evident that at least one or two dimensions form the core issues defining the adolescent-parent cultural gap.

For instance, if the parents are *past-oriented* in the time dimension (as are most parents from traditional cultures, such as Asian and Hispanic cultures), they will naturally insist on "the way we do it, the way your grandparents did it." Hence, "no tattoos," "no blue hair," "no pierced tongues," "no drugs," "home by 10:00 P.M." By contrast, an adolescent may be *present-oriented* (as most adolescents are) and is therefore more inclined to be influenced by peers, or at least pressured to conform to contemporary peer values. Hence, "tattoos," "blue hair," "pierced tongues," "drugs," and "home next morning, if at all." By providing the adolescents and their parents with a model that enables them to identify core issues and supplies them with a language for talking about these issues, the value-orientation model may be a vehicle by which they can begin to negotiate their cultural gaps and develop more therapeutic compromises. A more detailed presentation of the clinical use of the value-orientation model in clinical work with adolescents has been published elsewhere (Ponce 1995).

Immigration, Minority, and Ethnic Identity Issues

Immigrant adolescents from cultures in which they were considered "grown-up" and assumed adult responsibilities will predictably experience major acculturation problems, including significant "psychopathologies," reminiscent of those of the adolescent refugees in the 1970s and 1980s from war-torn Southeast Asian countries, such as Vietnam, Cambodia, and Laos, who were relocated to North American and European countries (Messer and Rasmussen 1986; Nguyen and Williams 1989). Psychotherapy with these adolescents and their significant others (parents, legal custodians, adoptive parents) will require a lot of psychoeducational work, particularly if the adoptive parents or legal custodians are from another culture, because the adolescents' "psychopathologies" could very easily be misinterpreted and misunderstood. The thrust of the psychoeducational intervention is to understand the core issue, which is that these adolescents are forced to regress to a more dependent and childish status in the host society after having functioned as adults in their home societies prior to migration.

Psychotherapy with these adolescents, as well as with other so-called minority adolescents (it is becoming more and more difficult to find true minority groups in the United States, since it is fast becoming a "multicultural society"; see Iyer 1993), is probably best approached using Auerswald's (1986) "Poker-Bridge" thought experiment model. Auerswald, one of the pioneers of the family therapy movement, would have us perform a "thought experiment" in which the question posed is, What would happen if you have four persons locked in a room where only a table and four chairs are present and on top of the table is a deck of playing cards? Two of the persons *only* know how to play poker and, further, are absolutely convinced that poker is the *only* game played with cards. The same conditions apply to the remaining two, except they only know how to play bridge. In a very clever and ingenious way, Auerswald then proceeds to outline various responses that could be profitably used to understand the dilemmas and conflicts two groups undergo who are aware only of the "game" they happen to know (substitute "culture" or "ethnicity" for "game," and the two groups of players for "minorities" versus "mainstream" cultures). More important, the model provides various ways of resolving the conflicts—in effect, ways of successful "acculturation." For instance, the poker player (immigrants, minorities, adolescents) could learn how to play bridge (mainstream culture, majority, parents) once there is recognition that there are actually two *different* games going on, and vice versa.

Conclusion

It was the basic premise of this chapter that in order to do effective culture-responsive psychotherapy with adolescents, the therapist must be not only sensitive but also *responsive* to factors in the adolescent, himself or herself, and the psychotherapeutic process. Culture constitutes the overarching context that provides meaning, purpose, and direction to the therapist's and the adolescent's therapeutic activities. In other words, there are specific *competencies* that must be recognized and learned if one is to be successful or, at a bare minimum, to do no harm in providing psychotherapeutic services to youngsters from different cultures. In terms of *knowledge* base, the therapist must be aware of the impact of developmental substages and psychosocial factors such as fragmentation of the family, rapid technological advances, drugs, youth gangs, and so forth on the overall therapeutic process. *Attitudinally,* the therapist must be open to exploring factors in himself or herself that could ease and facilitate, or hinder and make difficult, working with youngsters from a different culture. In particular, the therapist ought to be familiar with his or her clinical worldviews and how these direct him or her to behave in certain peculiar and predictable ways in transactions with adolescent patients.

In addition, specific *skills* are needed: the ability to establish clear, relevant, and helpful therapeutic contracts; use his or her understanding of the different therapeutic phases effectively; use his or her appreciation of a continuum of psychotherapeutic styles as a basis for effecting successful therapeutic fits or matches; and mobilize set (e.g., the therapist's use of his or her appreciation of the various worldviews of the key people involved, to effect therapeutic changes) and setting (e.g., consciously factoring in where therapy occurs to achieve maximum results—office? mall? beach? McDonald's) forces to achieve therapeutic goals.

In conclusion, we know that Hispanics and Asians are rapidly and profoundly altering the demographic profile of the United States (Iyer 1993; "The New America" *U.S. News & World Report* 1995), making culture a very important and urgent consideration in whatever we are planning to do—which, in our specific case, is to conduct cross-cultural psychotherapy with adolescents. To the clinician and practicing therapist, the implication is clear: like it or not, it is no longer sufficient to be competent clinically; one must also be a clinically culture-responsive "anthropologist" (Canino and Spurlock 1994).

References

Ariès P: Centuries of Childhood: A Social History of Family Life. Translated by Baldick R. London, Jonathan Cape, 1961

Auerswald E: Family therapy as a movement: epistemological barriers to ontological freedom. Journal of Strategic and Systemic Therapies 5:14–19, 1986

Bergin AE: The evaluation of treatment outcomes, in Handbook of Psychotherapy and Behavior Change. Edited by Bergin AE, Garfield S. New York, Wiley, 1971, pp 34–46

Canino I, Spurlock J: Culturally Diverse Children and Adolescents: Assessments, Diagnosis, and Treatment. New York, Guilford, 1994

Char W, Tseng W, Lum K, et al: The Chinese, in People and Cultures of Hawaii. Edited by McDermott JF Jr, Tseng WS, Maretzki TW. Honolulu, University of Hawaii Press, 1980, pp 53–72

Demos J, Demos V: Adolescence in historical perspective. Journal of Marriage and the Family 31:632–638, 1969

Frank J: Persuasion and Healing: A Comparative Study of Psychotherapy, 3rd Edition. Baltimore, MD, Johns Hopkins University Press, 1991

Geraty R, Hendren R, Flaa C: Ethical perspectives on managed care as it relates to child and adolescent psychiatry. J Am Acad Child Adolesc Psychiatry 31:398–402, 1992

Iyer P: The global village finally arrives, in The New Face of America: How Immigrants are Shaping the World's First Multicultural Society. Time 142(21):86–87, 1993

Kluckhohn F, Strodtbeck C: Variations in Value Orientations. New York, Peterson and Row, 1961

McLuhan M: War and Peace in the Global Village. New York, McGraw-Hill, 1968

Messer M, Rasmussen N: Southeast Asian children in America: the impact of change. Pediatrics 78:323–329, 1986

The New America. U.S. News & World Report, July 10, 1995

Nguyen N, Williams H: Transition from East to West: Vietnamese adolescents and their parents. J Am Acad Child Adolesc Psychiatry 28:505–515, 1989

Offer D, Schonert-Reichl K: Debunking the myths of adolescence: findings from recent research. J Am Acad Child Adolesc Psychiatry 31:1003–1014, 1992

Ponce D: Extramarital affairs: meaning and impact on the Filipino immigrant family. Filipinas: Journal of Philippine Studies 7:1–10, 1986

Ponce D: Erotic countertransference issues in a residential treatment center. Journal of Residential Treatment Center for Children and Youth 11:107–123, 1993

Ponce D: Value orientation: clinical applications. Journal of Residential Treatment Center for Children and Youth 12:29–42, 1995

Potter L, Rosenberg M, Hammond R, et al: Suicide in youth: a public health framework. J Am Acad Child Adolesc Psychiatry 37:484–487, 1998

Russell R: Reassessing Psychotherapy Research. New York, Guilford, 1994

Shafer M, Irwin C: The adolescent patient, in Pediatrics, 19th Edition. Edited by Rudolph A. New York, Appleton & Lange, 1991, pp 39–81

Taffel R: The second family. The Family Therapy Networker 20(3):36–45, 1996

Vargas LA, Koss-Chioino JD (eds): Working With Culture: Psychotherapeutic Interventions With Ethnic Minority Children and Adolescents. San Francisco, CA, Jossey-Bass, 1992

CHAPTER 14

The Ethnic Minority Elderly

F. M. Baker, M.D., M.P.H., F.A.P.A.
Junji Takeshita, M.D.

In the United States, four broad categories of ethnicity have been officially identified as minorities: African Americans, American Indians and Alaskan natives, Asian Americans and Pacific Islanders, and Hispanic Americans. Although, in reality, there are at least three groups within the category of Americans of African origin, more than 250 recognized Native American tribes, at least 17 different ethnic groups among Asian Americans and Pacific Islanders, and at least six different groups composing Hispanic Americans, these four broad categories are used for convenience by government agencies (Baker 2000; Baker and Lightfoot 1993).

By the year 2050, ethnic minority elderly will make up more than one-fifth of the total United States population—a trend deserving of mental health workers' attention (Angel and Hogan 1991). Despite the increase in the proportion of this population, they will continue to exist as a "double minority." They not only will have minority status from an ethnic perspective but also may be culturally underprivileged because of their age. This is a subgroup that tends to underutilize mental health facilities and the treatment modality of psychotherapy and therefore needs special concern and care.

Case Vignettes

Mrs. Arnold

Mrs. Arnold, an 82-year-old, widowed African American woman, was brought to the therapist's office by a niece who is her primary companion. The niece, appearing somewhat embarrassed, reported that Mrs. Arnold was increasingly confused, had begun to misplace items, and was less interested in her correspondence with friends and former students. Mrs. Arnold had begun to lose weight, and recently she mixed up her medications for hypertension and congestive heart failure.

After an evaluation, including communication with her internist, the therapist found that Mrs. Arnold had no prior history of memory problems and remained an active, respected leader in her community and in her church. The relocation of her three children to other states because of promotions in their careers caused her some distress, particularly with the loss of contact with her grandchildren. Her symptoms had developed over the 6 months since their move and were consistent with a major depressive disorder.

Although Mrs. Arnold had never been to a psychiatrist, she wondered whether she would have "to lie on a couch for 5 years and talk you [the therapist] to death." Providing information about the illness of depression and its treatment, the therapist recognized her level of sophistication (retired university biology teacher) and enabled her to maintain her sense of competence, while acknowledging an illness of the mind—something potentially very threatening to her sense of self-definition and mastery.

Mrs. Arnold felt comfortable with her therapist, a 38-year-old African American man whom she viewed as one of her successful "students." The therapist had to avoid viewing Mrs. Arnold as a maternal figure. The age difference between the patient and her therapist facilitated an exploration of feelings about the children who had "abandoned" her. Focusing on her prior successful coping capacities in a life review (e.g., only African American doctoral candidate in a white northeastern school, early widow with three children, successful negotiation of the academic career ladder), Mrs. Arnold was able to reflect on her current situation and identify the opportunities within it.

A weekly telephone visit with her grandchildren and the establishment of an after-school program at her church for the working parents of her community provided the contact with the next generation that she sought and valued. In treatment, she identified her expectation that she would remain the geographic, as well as the spiritual, center of her family. Mobilizing her coping capacities facilitated her creation of a new role within her church, which fulfilled her psychological need and aided the young parents and children of her community.

Discussion

The case above illustrates several issues in the psychotherapy of minority elderly persons. Having a therapist of the same ethnicity assisted in transference issues, but the clinician had to be alert to the potential pitfalls of a maternal countertransference. The use of a life review to identify strengths and prior successful coping capacities was helpful in this case, and would have been even more so if the patient's cultural background differed from that of the therapist. There often exists a wide diversity among the different birth cohorts of the elderly of an ethnic minority group in terms of their educational level and orientation to psychotherapy. These factors need to be assessed with each older person. There was an absence of stigma for psychotherapy for this educated African American woman.

Mr. Running Bear

Mr. Running Bear, a 62-year-old, married Navajo man, had lived near the New Mexico tribal reservation for 30 years. He was a skilled craftsman, recognized as a major artist in Navajo turquoise jewelry making. He had residual left-sided weakness from a stroke that he had suffered 1 year previously. He remained able to use his dominant right hand.

Mr. Running Bear recognized that over the past 4 months his ability to conceptualize designs had been affected. He believed a Navajo religious ceremony (a sing) held 1 year earlier had been very helpful in limiting the severity of his poststroke deficits, but there was concern that there may be a new illness. Although he spent time in the sweat lodge to help him regain harmony with his environment, his symptoms remained. Reluctantly, he acknowledged thinking increasingly of death.

His (Navajo) medicine man recommended that he continue his visits to the sweat lodge and prepared a special herbal medication for his consumption. He informed Mr. Running Bear that if his symptoms persisted after this treatment, he should visit the (Western) clinic's physician, with whom the medicine man had developed a relationship of mutual respect over the years. Eventually, Mr. Running Bear was referred by the clinic's physician to a Caucasian psychiatrist. This therapist acknowledged Mr. Running Bear's need to regain harmony with his environment. Supporting his continued work with the Navajo medicine man, the therapist explained to Mr. Running Bear that there was medicine that could relieve his symptoms. The therapist also recommended regular visits to talk about not only the medicine but also other things of concern in his life. Mr. Running Bear, with the support of his family, agreed to take advantage of working with both his native healer and the Western therapist.

During the course of therapy, Mr. Running Bear identified his anger and sense of loss of his cultural heritage caused by his placement in an Indian boarding school at age 12. He reflected that his Navajo identity had to be regained as an adult. He feared that the loss of his skill as a Navajo jeweler would cause him to lose his cultural identity again. Although familiar with Navajo culture, the Caucasian therapist was careful to avoid apologizing or rationalizing the decision of the Indian Health Service to acculturate Indian adolescents by placing them in boarding schools. The ethnicity of the therapist facilitated Mr. Running Bear's opportunity to work through his anger toward American society. At the end of treatment, Mr. Running Bear began a special lodge for elders who had also been placed in Indian boarding schools during their adolescent years to talk about and express their feelings.

Discussion

This case illustrates a pragmatic approach, not only by the patient but also by his health care providers. Rather than focusing on a dichotomous model of either Western medicine or native healing, the therapist and healers wisely took advantage of both systems. The case also illustrates that, even for the elderly, unresolved issues from earlier life stages may be identified and worked through in therapy. In this case, the Caucasian therapist used the patient's own negative ethnic transference to facilitate the working through of his unresolved feelings of anger and the identity and role confusion that resulted from his forceful separation from his family of origin. With identification and mobilization of his affects, the patient was able to effectively mourn his lost Navajo adolescence and to recognize the strengths that had enabled him to survive and to succeed in both cultures.

Mrs. Tanabe

Mrs. Tanabe, an 80-year-old woman of Japanese ancestry, was brought to a psychiatrist for depressive symptoms and mild dementia. She was living with her eldest son, Robert, who was also retired. Mrs. Tanabe was a member of the so-called *kibei* group, born in Hawaii but sent by her parents back to Japan for education, returning to the United States as a young adult. Although she had lived in the United States for most of her adult life, she spoke primarily Japanese. Her English was rather limited, even in daily conversation. Her four children, including Robert, spoke almost no Japanese.

Mrs. Tanabe was relieved to learn that her therapist happened to speak Japanese. She tearfully acknowledged her frustration in communicating with her children, particularly after her husband died several years ago. The therapist noted that, during a joint session with Mrs. Tanabe and her son Robert, he kept addressing his mother as *okusan,* a Japanese word meaning "wife," rather than *okasan,* meaning "mother."

It became apparent that the son could no longer care for his mother because of her progressing frailty. But Mrs. Tanabe was strongly resistant to being placed in a public care facility. To her, this meant her family was abandoning her, the worst thing that could happen. The therapist assisted the son in helping his mother change her view and accept the suggested placement. Finally, Mrs. Tanabe went to a nursing home, where she was pleased to find other elderly residents who spoke Japanese.

Discussion

In this case, psychotherapy involved several aspects, including psychoeducation, family therapy, and supportive therapy. This case demonstrates that language can be a serious obstacle to communication between the elderly and their adult children, contributing significantly to the development of depression in an aged parent. The therapist facilitated the communication between mother and son by serving not only as a translator but also as a broker for the cultural gap that existed between them.

Issues in Psychotherapy

Entry Into Treatment

The aged ethnic minority patient is usually brought to the therapist by the family and commonly views mental illness as shameful (Baker 1990). Therefore, seeing a mental health professional may be a frightening and anxiety-provoking experience in itself. The presence of family members or members of the elder's religious community can place the elder more at ease and ameliorate some of this distress. Recognition of and attention to the cultural expectations of "seeing the doctor," acknowledging the role of the family in facilitating and negotiating treatment for the elder, and educating the patient to the purpose and methods of the "talking treatment"—all contribute to the successful outcome of the psychotherapeutic process.

Initially, the minority elder may be interviewed with the elder's spouse or sibling of the same age to obtain information about the family's decision to bring the elder for help. The older person should be seen individually, even if he or she is very reluctant. In addition to the basic tenet of interviewing the identified patient to obtain a direct history, it is important to respect the unique role of the minority elder in the elder's family and to acknowledge that role in the interview. Such awareness on the part of the evaluating therapist can decrease some of the stress and anxiety experienced by the minority elder as a reluctant psychiatric patient.

Educational level, prior experience with the health care system, impressions of the field of psychiatry, cultural attitudes toward mental illness, and expectations of the health care professional are some of the factors affecting the participation of the minority elder in psychotherapy (Ahmed 1997; American Psychiatric Association 1994; Baker 2000). These factors need to be explored and managed from the very beginning to facilitate the development of a successful therapeutic alliance.

New Immigrants

New immigrants face issues of adjusting to a new home, developing an understanding of a new culture, and sometimes learning a new language. Although many older immigrants did not complete a high school education, some 25% of older Asian Americans did complete high school and further education (Baker and Lightfoot 1993). It is important for the therapist to clarify the prior experiences of the elder, including education, experiences of trauma, work history, level of acculturation, and language fluency.

American-Born Ethnic Minority Elders

American-born ethnic minority elders have different issues in entering treatment. Acculturation and language fluency are not a concern. A therapist may erroneously assume that a minority elder still has values from the home country. It is important to acknowledge that this group has struggled with the effects of American racism and prejudice over a life span. Although the four broad categories of ethnic minority elders are very diverse, they share the common experience of having suffered exclusion and negative labeling by American society during some period (Baker 1982, 1987). Examples of such exclusion and negative labeling are the legalized segregation of African Americans and the Asian Exclusion Acts and "Yellow Peril" headlines in the newspapers of the early 1900s (Baker 2000). Such factors may have been more significant in the formative years of adolescence and early adulthood of these American-born minority elders.

Elders of minority ethnicity who suffered discrimination during adolescence and early adulthood may mistrust a Caucasian therapist and may prefer to see a therapist of the same ethnicity. Varying reactions to the dominant culture have been reported for Asian American elders (American Psychiatric Association 1994). These reactions range from identification with the aggressor through devaluation of the elder's culture and values to a healthy acceptance of the elder's cultural background. It is important to establish whether a second- or third-generation American-born minority elder continues to cling to old values and traditions from the home country that are no longer practiced there (Bernal and Gutierrez 1988; Hughes 1993; Jimenez and de Figueiredo 1994; Sakauye and Chacko 1994). For example, elderly Japanese Americans may continue to practice various traditions and customs that are no longer practiced in modern-day Japan.

Engagement

Minority elders often expect that the therapist, if a physician, will do something "medical" to the patient, such as checking the patient's pulse and blood pressure or listening to the heart and lungs. In some Asian cultures, the more experienced the healer, the fewer questions are asked (Chien and Yamamoto 1982; Sakauye and Chacko 1994). Thus, minority elder patients may expect a very focused interview, emphasizing the physical examination. It is important for the therapist to be aware of these potential expectations, even if the treatment is psychotherapy. An exhaustive, detailed history reassuring to a minority elder with an orientation to and familiarity with Western medicine may, to another minority elder, be clear evidence of the incompetence of the physician (Chien and Yamamoto 1982; Sakauye and Chacko 1994).

It is important for the therapist to listen to the elder's description of the illness and what he or she expects to gain from the visit. Communication can be greatly facilitated if the evaluating therapist can speak of the diagnosed illness in terms that recognize the elder's cultural conceptualization of the specific symptoms experienced (Acosta et al. 1982; Baker 1995; Bernal and Gutierrez 1988; Shore and Manson 1981).

The older patient may be hesitant to respond directly to questions.

Looking the therapist in the eye and speaking spontaneously about personal matters, particularly in front of younger family members, may be considered socially inappropriate behavior (Clevenger 1982; Thompson 1994). Such knowledge will prevent a social gaffe by the therapist, which may alienate the minority elder (Chien and Yamamoto 1982).

Transference

Depending on the age of the therapist, the minority elder may view the therapist as a successful and favored child or an extended family member, if the transference is a positive one. This will facilitate the initial engagement of the minority elder in therapy. However, it will be necessary to move the transference away from an extended family member and more toward a concerned, informed community member to enable the ethnic minority elder to be comfortable in revealing experiences that the elder may view as embarrassing.

If the therapist, by ethnic background, language, or nonverbal behavior, reminds the minority elder of persons who discriminated against or verbally assaulted him or her, or persons who were present at the time of a traumatic event that the elder experienced, the initial transference will be negative. Awareness of the elder's life history in the context of larger societal events (Asnes 1983; Baker 1994; Baker and Lightfoot 1993) will enable the therapist to interpret the ethnic transference and demonstrate an appreciation of the difficulties that the minority elder has survived. In situations in which a therapist of similar ethnic and cultural background is available, and the elder has significant difficulty with the treating therapist, a referral may be the most facilitating intervention that the therapist can make. When no alternative therapist is available, participation in community groups at senior centers or at the elder's religious institution will provide age-cohort peers who have had similar life experiences. The support of such a group and, if necessary, referral to the elder's family physician for supportive therapy and medication management may be the most appropriate intervention, if the negative transference cannot be resolved.

Potentially, therapists of any ethnic background can work effectively with any ethnic minority elder. What is required is a willingness to understand the culture, to learn the history of the specific ethnic group, and to have members of one's staff or treatment team who are fluent in the language of the elder. If the ethnic minority elder is monolingual in a language that the therapist cannot speak, and there is no member of the treatment team who can complete the indicated psychotherapeutic work, referral to an appropriate therapist would be indicated.

Countertransference

Each therapist must remain sensitive to the specific circumstances or situations that will increase the probability for countertransference—both personal and ethnic. Working with older persons may stimulate a parental or mentor countertransference. Recognition of this risk should facilitate early identification and resolution through clarification of its etiology (Hughes 1993). Other countertransferences may occur, including the identification of the older patient as a representative of a former wartime enemy, resulting in a negative (ethnic) countertransference based on the therapist's prior acculturation. Identification of the source of the negative and/or rejecting feelings toward the minority elder will enable the therapist to regain a neutral stance.

Family and Community

The importance of working with the family and the minority elder's community (including native healers) has been illustrated by the therapies for Mrs. Arnold and Mr. Running Bear described earlier in this chapter. The family therapy may involve education about the elder's illness, support, or resolution of unresolved issues, such as traumatic life experiences, acculturation, and conflict in role expectations. Thus, psychotherapy may involve multiple levels (Acosta and Evans 1982; American Psychiatric Association 1994; Baker and Lightfoot 1993; Bernal and Gutierrez 1988). Use of family therapy with ethnic minority elders can be particularly effective because of the emphasis of these diverse ethnic minority groups on the importance of family and community ties (Taylor 1985). In the same context, group psychotherapy with minority elders may provide an age-cohort reference group, provide a forum for the sharing of common experiences, acknowledge survival through adversity, and facilitate group members' coming to terms with having a mental illness and understanding how talking therapy can help in ameliorating their symptoms.

Attitudes Toward Getting Old

Although people around the world share universal views about aging, there are certain cultural variations in attitudes toward getting old, on a spectrum of positive to negative. There also may be a difference between the cultural ideal and the actual experience of the elderly. For instance, the American therapist may tend to idealize the aging process in Japan, viewing the elderly as greatly respected and cared for and faring much better than the elderly in

Western cultures (Tobin 1987). As a result, a therapist may be blind to obvious signs of neglect or abuse, such as malnutrition.

The attitude of therapeutic nihilism that may be present in the elderly can be compounded in the ethnic minority patient. In fact, a similar attitude may be present in the therapist. Clinicians need to understand that, regardless of ethnicity, an elder may be capable of benefiting from psychotherapy, particularly if the therapist expresses positive value for the patient's cultural heritage.

Relationships With Adult Children

Many elderly live with or are cared for by adult children, who may be approaching the age of retirement themselves. Other caregivers may include grandchildren or other relatives. Although extended families are a source of support, the close contact can also spark new problems deriving from old family conflicts. There often exist wide cultural gaps between the elderly parents and their children because of remarkably different life experiences encountered by the separate generations (American Psychiatric Association 1994). These gaps can be a source of stress and conflict. The challenge in therapy is how to help the elder communicate with the offspring who have acculturated differently (as shown in the case of Mrs. Tanabe described earlier in this chapter).

Death and Dying

The aging process involves illness and inevitable death. Death is a natural phenomenon, part of the circle of life, but the subject of death is not commonly faced or easily discussed in many societies. In some cultures, it is even considered taboo to mention death. From the psychological standpoint, however, many elders are comfortable with death, particularly in comparison with younger individuals. When a therapist is working with a dying patient, cultural factors may be the key to resolving the practical arrangements that can be so troublesome for the family.

Suggestions

Psychotherapy with ethnic minority elders may be particularly complicated. Sociocultural factors such as race, ethnicity, religion, language, country of origin, modern versus traditional values, immigration, socioeconomic status, perception of minority status in the United States and in the country of origin, and educational level affect the elder's self-definition and ability to participate in psychotherapy. Age-specific multiple medical illnesses and impaired cognitive function may play a more important role than culture for some ethnic elders in determining the most appropriate form of psychotherapy for them. Although aging is a universal process, the adaptations and methods of coping with the aging process are influenced by culture.

In working with the ethnic minority elder, the following are important considerations:

1. *Begin by obtaining the needed life history (work, marriage, children, countries of residence) and education of the patient.* Is the elder a new immigrant to the United States, or is the elder a third-generation, American-born college graduate who is a retired attorney?
2. *Clarify the specific major life events of the minority elder.* Has the elder survived a war or military action in his or her country of origin? Is the American-born minority elder frightened of being mugged, because of the change in the community in which the elder has lived for over 30 years?
3. *Involve the person who accompanies the minority elder in the initial interview in order to establish the social support network for the minority elder.* Is the elder the "emotional and spiritual center" of the family? Or is the elder isolated and alone because, in the case of Asian Americans, the Asian Exclusion Acts of the early 1900s prevented the elder from bringing family members to the United States?
4. *Explore the elder's definition of illness and the person(s) and settings that the elder identifies as being helpful in treating his or her specific symptoms.* How does the minority elder view an illness of the mind? Are there words in the minority elder's language for "depression" or "dementia"? What words does the minority elder use to describe the symptoms experienced?
5. *Be sensitive to the nonverbal behavior of the minority elder, particularly when the elder is seen alone.* For example, the therapist should recognize that avoiding eye-contact and answering rather than initiating conversation may be evidence of respect for the physician rather than withdrawal due to depressive illness.
6. *Clarify what the elder expects to gain from talking with the therapist.* Is the therapist expected to prescribe a pill, to see the elder again in a month versus a week, or to have the patient's vital signs checked at each visit?
7. *Explain the range of treatments for the symptoms experienced by the elder.* Treatment may include physical examination, education about the ill-

ness, information about the various treatments available, and expected outcome of treatment. These explanations should be tailored to the understanding of the minority elder and the accompanying family member. The therapist may outline, if appropriate, a specific, desired plan of treatment, mentioning the other options that are not appropriate for this specific elder.

8. *Acknowledge that alternatives to Western medicine are used by many people and explore with the minority elder whether he or she is in concurrent treatment with an acupuncturist, an herbalist, a root doctor, a spiritual leader, or a medicine man.* The minority elder should be encouraged to describe both traditional and Western medicines being used and that have been effective in the past. This will enable the minority elder to make maximum use of all health providers and the therapist to identify potential drug-drug interactions should psychoactive medications be prescribed.

9. *Consider using a life review format within the therapy.* Incorporation of a life review format within the therapy can facilitate the identification of successful coping strategies used by the elder in the past, as well as potential areas of unresolved conflicts or repressed traumatic events.

10. *Consider incorporating family meetings within the course of therapy.* Because of the importance of family and extended family for many minority elders, incorporating family meetings within the course of therapy can facilitate treatment by providing an additional perspective on how the minority elder is functioning, as well as providing a forum for resolving and clarifying areas of conflict.

11. *Establish the psychological, personal, and practical resources of the minority elder.* Identifying these resourcs will aid the therapist in choosing the most appropriate interventions. Interventions might include individual, family, or group psychotherapy, or a combination of these over the course of treatment.

12. *Clarify the social support network of the minority elder (extended family, community groups, religious community).* Such clarification can be an effective technique to facilitate the initial evaluation and to continue the treatment process. Although some ethnic minority elders may be unfamiliar with and initially hostile to psychotherapy, an experience with "talking treatment"—particularly when sanctioned by family members and a native healer—can successfully involve the elder in a new form of treatment that can improve the elder's symptoms and quality of life.

References

Acosta FX, Evans LA: The Hispanic-American patient, in Psychotherapy for Low-Income and Minority Patients. Edited by Acosta FX, Yamamoto J. Evans LA. New York, Plenum, 1982, pp 51–82

Acosta FX, Yamamoto J, Evans LA: Psychotherapy for Low-Income and Minority Patients. New York, Plenum, 1982

Ahmed I: Geriatric psychopathology, in Culture and Psychopathology: A Guide to Clinical Assessment. Edited by Tseng WS, Streltzer J. New York, Brunner/Mazel, 1997, pp 223–240

American Psychiatric Association, Task Force on Ethnic Minority Elderly: Ethnic Minority Elderly: A Task Force Report. Washington, DC, American Psychiatric Association, 1994

Angel JL, Hogan DP: The demography of minority aging populations, in Minority Elders: Longevity, Economics, and Health: Building a Public Policy Base. Edited by Harootyan LK. Washington, DC, Gerontological Society of America, 1991, pp 1–13

Asnes DP: Psychotherapy of the elderly: the life validation approach in psychotherapy with elderly patients. J Geriatr Psychiatry 16:87–97, 1983

Baker FM: The black elderly: biopsychosocial perspective within an age cohort and adult development context. J Geriatr Psychiatry 14:225–239, 1982

Baker FM: The Afro-American life cycle: success, failure, and mental health. J Natl Med Assoc 79:625–633, 1987

Baker FM: Ethnic minority elderly: differential diagnosis, medication, treatment, and outcomes, in Minority Aging: Essential Curricula Content for Selected Health and Allied Health Professions (DHHS Publ No HRS P-V-90-4). Edited by Harper MS. Washington, DC, U.S. Department of Health and Human Services, 1990, pp 549–577

Baker FM: Psychiatric treatment of older African Americans. Hospital and Community Psychiatry 45:32–37, 1994

Baker FM: Mental health issues in elderly African Americans. Clin Geriatr Med 11:1–13, 1995

Baker FM: Minority issues in geriatric psychiatry, in Comprehensive Textbook of Psychiatry/VII, 7th Edition. Edited by Sadock BJ, Sadock VA. Baltimore, MD, Lippincott Williams & Wilkins, 2000

Baker FM, Lightfoot OB: Psychiatric care of ethnic elders, in Culture, Ethnicity, and Mental Illness. Edited by Gaw AC. Washington, DC, American Psychiatric Press, 1993, pp 517–522

Bernal G, Gutierrez M: Cubans, in Clinical Guidelines in Cross-Cultural Mental Health. Edited by Comas-Diaz L, Griffith EEH. New York, Wiley, 1988, pp 233–261

Chien C, Yamamoto J: Asian-Americans and Pacific Islanders, in Effective Psycho-therapy for Low-Income and Minority Patients. Edited by Acosta FX, Yamamoto J, Evans LA. New York, Plenum, 1982, pp 117–145

Clevenger J: Native Americans, in Cross-Cultural Psychiatry. Edited by Gaw AC. Boston, MA, John Wright, 1982, pp 149–158

Hughes CC: Culture in clinical psychiatry, in Culture, Ethnicity, and Mental Illness. Edited by Gaw AC. Washington, DC, American Psychiatric Press, 1993, pp 3–41

Jimenez RG, de Figueiredo JM: Issues in the psychiatric care of Hispanic American elders, in Ethnic Minority Elderly: A Task Force Report. Washington, DC, American Psychiatric Association, 1994, pp 63–89

Sakauye KM, Chacko RC: Issues in the psychiatric care of Asian/Pacific American elders, in Ethnic Minority Elderly: A Task Force Report of the American Psychiatric Association. Washington, DC, American Psychiatric Association, 1994, pp 115–147

Shore JH, Manson SM: Cross-cultural studies of depression among American Indians and Alaska Natives. White Cloud Journal 2(2):5–12, 1981

Taylor RJ: The extended family as a source of support to elderly blacks. Gerontologist 25:488–495, 1985

Thompson JW: Issues in the psychiatric care of American Indian and Alaska Native elders, in Ethnic Minority Elderly: A Task Force Report. Washington, DC, American Psychiatric Association, 1994, pp 91–113

Tobin JJ: The American idealization of old age in Japan. Gerontologist 27:53–58, 1987

PART 5

Special Models of Therapy

CHAPTER 15

Marital Therapy for Intercultural Couples

Jing Hsu, M.D.

The term *intercultural marriage* refers to marriages formed by partners with relatively diverse cultural backgrounds. They may be addressed simply as "intermarried couples" or "intercultural couples." An intercultural marriage is not the same thing as an interracial marriage, which may involve greater or lesser differences in terms of cultural background. *Culture* is defined as a lifestyle with unique beliefs, values, and behaviors, and it is often associated with race, ethnicity, religion, and other factors. It generally is recognized that the numbers of interracial and intercultural marriages are increasing in the United States.

Intermarried couples have a greater likelihood of encountering problems because of different views, beliefs, value systems, attitudes, and habits than couples who are of similar cultures or intraculturally married couples (the latter referred to as "intramarried couples") (Kitano et al. 1984). Cultural factors often play a crucial role in therapy involving such couples (Solsberry 1994) and, therefore, warrant the therapist's special attention and consideration. Clearly, the fact that each partner is from a different culture does not in and of itself mean that a couple's relationship is unsatisfactory. However, when an intercultural couple is having difficulty, paying special attention to cultural aspects of the relationship will often bear fruit.

Case Vignettes

Mary and Kalani

A Caucasian, middle-aged woman, Mary, came to a psychiatric clinic seeking help. She complained that she was feeling depressed, lost, and lonely, as she and her husband, a Hawaiian named Kalani, were on the verge of breaking up.

The couple had married 2 years before, shortly after Mary's divorce from her previous husband, a Caucasian. Mary's parents had felt that the ethnic and racial differences between Mary and Kalani would have a negative effect on the marriage. Mary recalled a time, prior to the marriage, when she had placed her fair-skinned arm over Kalani's dark-skinned one and announced to her parents that even though she and Kalani had different skin colors, that would not interfere with their abiding love for each other. Kalani, too, reflected the same optimism when he assured Mary's parents that his wide and varied cultural experiences around the world while in the military had prepared him for a successful marriage to Mary.

When Mary and her two teenage daughters from her previous marriage moved with Kalani to Hawaii, they were warmly welcomed by Kalani's family. However, the initial excitement and good feelings did not last very long. Soon, Mary would become upset when, every weekend, Kalani would visit his parents. Mary felt that this time should be spent with "his own family"— Mary and the girls—as a family unit. Kalani, on the other hand, felt that, because he had spent many years away from his family of origin, he was obliged to make up for lost time with them. Kalani argued that, according to Hawaiian cultural tradition, not only Mary and the two kids but also his parents, siblings, and other relatives were part of his "own" family, his "large" family. He felt that, as a Hawaiian, he was expected to be with his "large" family as much as he could. To do otherwise would be to insult the "whole family."

Initially, despite her reluctance, Mary and her daughters would go with Kalani each weekend to visit with his family of origin. However, as time passed, she found herself unable to adapt to many of the Hawaiian ways of life. For example, she would express her frank opinions at family gatherings. This embarrassed and distressed Kalani, who, along with the other members of his family, considered such behavior impolite and aggressive. It was considered bad manners (and an evil sign) for a female hen to crow. Kalani had stressed to Mary, prior to moving to Hawaii, that she should "walk soft" in his parents' house, so as not to offend anybody. Mary, however, had no idea what walking softly entailed.

Upon learning that her in-laws were unhappy with her behavior, Mary was so upset that she left Kalani's parents' house one day without a word of good-bye. Mary was completely unaware of the prevailing Hawaiian custom that if one leaves a house without a proper "good-bye" to the master of the house, then that person would no longer be welcome at the house. As a result of this unfortunate intercultural transaction, Mary was no longer invited to Kalani's parents' house. Kalani continued to visit, while Mary stayed home alone.

There were also problems at home. Mary's two daughters, like many teenagers, enjoyed warm and boisterous talking at the dinner table. Mary encouraged this behavior as developing a "closeness" among the family members. Kalani, on the other hand, was very annoyed. His feeling, based on his Hawaiian upbringing, was that children should not make noise during meals—that they should "be seen but not heard." Kalani preferred that the girls listen quietly to and learn from the "adult" conversation between him and Mary. Indeed, he was so disturbed by his stepdaughters' "misbehavior" that he physically punished them. For Kalani, this discipline was the same as that which he had received from his father by means of a leather belt. Mary was offended and upset by Kalani's behavior. Furthermore, she "could not bear to see" her daughters treated in such a "cruel way."

Mary, feeling that their marriage was on the verge of breaking up, asked Kalani to go with her for counseling. Kalani was extremely reluctant, insisting that any problems that the family had "should be taken care of at home." They did finally come in for therapy, but only after Mary threatened to leave if they did not seek help together.

Discussion

It is clear that this couple tried to deny from the very beginning the wide cultural gap that existed between them. It is also obvious that, in addition to personal factors, including the motivation for this marriage, cultural differences contributed significantly to the couple's marital problems. In therapy, the first thing the therapist did was to help the couple realize that "love" was not enough to keep them together. They needed to recognize the vast differences between them and work on them. Kalani was advised that to warn his wife to "walk softly" was not enough. She, as the newcomer in his home setting, needed detailed cultural guidance in how she should behave in his Hawaiian environment. She needed to have explained to her the meanings behind the cultural rules and the potential consequences if those rules were not observed.

Clarifying the definitions and meanings of the family and establishing family boundaries were issues that needed to be worked on in therapy as well. To what extent the couple needed to comply with each other's cultural expectations, and to what extent their own needs had to be considered, were the central issues that had to be examined and negotiated.

The therapist had to help the couple realize that many aspects of their cultural backgrounds were not only different from but opposite each other and that this could create serious consequences between them. For instance, children talking at dinnertime is considered a good thing in one culture but bad behavior in the other. On the whole, through therapy, they needed to learn not to insist on only *my* way (following *my* culture), but to examine the implications for *you* (according to *your* culture) and to search for solutions that allowed for compromise between the opposing positions, for the sake of *us,* the couple.

Maria and Andy

Maria, a Filipino woman, was brought to an emergency room by her Caucasian husband, Andy. Maria had taken an overdose of medication in response to a domestic incident that had occurred at home. After the acute medical crisis was over, Maria was discharged with the suggestion that she and Andy seek marital counseling together.

Maria had come to the United States by herself several years earlier for a college education and "a better life." Andy and Maria met each other at a bar and fell in love at first sight. Andy had previously dated several Caucasian women, but when he met Maria, he "knew right away that this was the kind of woman I wanted to marry." To him, Maria was passionate and subordinate and knew how to please a man.

They married in Maria's hometown in the Philippines. The wedding was a big celebration participated in by Maria's immediate family, other relatives, and her whole village. A young pig was killed and roasted, and the feast lasted for several days. Maria's family was very pleased that they now had an American as a son-in-law. Andy enjoyed the glorious reception that was given to him by all.

After the wedding, they returned to the United States. It was not too long before Maria began to receive mail and long-distance calls from her family in the Philippines. Much of it was requesting financial aid for various family matters—her mother needed money for her uncle's funeral, a niece was sick and needed money for hospitalization, and so on. In the beginning, Andy was happy to help her family. Shortly, though, he complained to Maria that he had married "her" and not her "family and relatives." Maria became distraught and tried to explain to Andy that if she did not respond to her family's requests for aid, then she would "lose face."

After they had been married a while, Maria became pregnant. Andy's sister chose the occasion to visit the couple. Maria was very excited to meet her sister-in-law for the first time. Tension arose at the airport when Andy suggested that his sister sit in the front seat and Maria in the back. Andy's intention was to provide a better view for his sister on her first visit to Hawaii, but he failed to explain the seating arrangement or the rationale to Maria beforehand. Maria construed the seating arrangement as a strong indication that Andy considered her "inferior" because she was not "white."

Upon arriving home, Andy directed Maria to commence dinner preparations while he made up the guest bed for his sister. This upset Maria again. She felt that it was her role, as the wife, to prepare the bed for any guest in their home—particularly for a female guest from her husband's family. Furthermore, Maria took this as an indication that Andy did not feel she was good enough or "worthy" to prepare a bed for his sister. She locked herself in the bathroom and swallowed all the pills in the medicine cabinet.

Discussion

Maria and Andy got along well as husband and wife until his or her family of origin was involved. This is a rather common phenomenon, even for intramarried couples. On these occasions, cultural rules come into play, and feelings are involved relating to the families of origin. These extramarital factors are severe when they involve cultural dimensions. The rules, expectations, and obligations demanded by a family of origin can be confusing, if not conflicting, for the couple.

In therapy, the strength and affinity that existed between the spouses were acknowledged from the very beginning, to enhance their hope of healing. The focus of therapy then concentrated on the problems relating to the families of origin. Andy was encouraged to communicate more effectively with Maria, explaining his "good" intentions and also obtaining his wife's consent, so that Maria's misinterpretations and suspicions (arising from her feeling of being treated as racially inferior) could be minimized or even avoided. For this couple, in spite of the dramatic crisis that occurred, the prognosis was reasonably optimistic after they learned through therapy how to communicate, understand, deal with, and resolve their differences in the future.

Common Problems Encountered by Intermarried Couples

Misguided Expectations Based on Projected Beliefs About Other Cultures

It has been speculated that some individuals who marry interracially have ulterior motives, such as rebelling against their families, being sexually curious about people of a different race, or seeking economic or class gains (Davidson 1992). Individuals often hold certain fantasies, beliefs, and stereotypes of other ethnic or cultural groups (Cohen 1982). These include, but are not limited to, traits and roles of the two genders. For instance, there is a common belief that Asian women are subservient to men and enjoy serving them. An often-related preconception is that Western men are romantic, fun-loving, and kind to their women. A Chinese wife might expect to be treated with consideration and respect, while her American husband might want to be pleased and served. The power of such beliefs may be a strong factor leading to interracial marriage.

After the marriage takes place, the couple may be troubled and disappointed if there is a gap between their fantasies and reality. This gap, based on ethnic projection and/or cultural stereotypes, can and often does create conflict, anger, and resentment. For example, in the case of Mary and Kalani presented earlier, Mary fantasized that, by marrying a Hawaiian husband, she could live a very relaxed and liberal life in Hawaii, without knowing that, in reality, she had to observe many cultural rules and the etiquette of her husband's Hawaiian family and community.

Shift in Implicit Ethnic/Racial Hierarchy

Individuals may view other ethnic or racial groups as either superior or inferior to their own. One may, consciously or unconsciously, marry someone from a supposedly inferior or superior group on the basis of his or her own personal needs, family dynamics, or practical concerns. This imbalance may be tolerated and even accepted by the "inferior" spouse when he or she marries a "superior" spouse. However, with time and growth, the "inferior" spouse may want a more egalitarian relationship. Such a desire for change from the tacit "initial contract" can result in marital conflict and distress. For example, Maria (in the case described earlier) was happy to marry "up" to a Caucasian husband, but, later, she became sensitive to any implication that she was a spouse of "inferior" ethnicity.

Difficulties in Communication

Very often, a major issue in intercultural marriage is language. When the partners' cultures do not share a common language, difficulties in communication can create great problems. Even if the partners can communicate in a common language, problems may still exist, particularly if the common language is not the native language of the partner(s). In such a situation, the communication between them is often rather superficial and limited. The meanings and feelings behind the words and between the lines are often not well communicated and understood, causing potential difficulties between the spouses, who need cognitive congruence for emotional closeness. This need is particularly true with regard to the subtle and delicate ways one "negotiates" relationship issues and expresses emotions.

Differences in Ways of Coping

Different cultures often have very different methods of coping with problems and resolving conflicts. For example, people from Asian cultures are more likely to use existing family or pseudo-family social systems to deal with crises, instead of professional or nonfamilial support systems. Kalani (in the case described earlier), following the Hawaiian way, chose to keep his complaints inside until they exploded. To communicate, to express and share feelings, and to apologize, if necessary, in order to resolve anger between the spouses—as Mary preferred to do—was not Kalani's way of dealing with crises that occurred between the couple. The two failed to resolve problems jointly in the same manner.

The case of Meilin and Tim illustrates two contrasting manners of coping.

> Meilin, a first-generation Chinese woman, married Tim, a fourth-generation American of European ancestry. When difficulties arose in their relationship, Meilin would often seek help by returning to her family of origin in Taiwan. In Chinese culture it is acceptable, and indeed expected, that a woman will seek temporary refuge from tensions in her marriage by returning to her parents' home and seeking guidance from them. Stereotypically, parents usually encourage the wife to return to her husband's home as soon as possible.

Tim, unaware of the norms of his wife's culture of origin, interpreted Meilin's behavior as "desertion" of her husband with the intent to separate or divorce. When Tim had emotional problems, he sought solace and advice outside his family. He discussed his marital problems with his golfing friends and the school counselor of the couple's child.

Once, after a particularly bitter physical argument between the two, Tim called the police. Meilin considered this public airing of their private problems to be Tim's attempt to publicly humiliate and discredit her, with the intention of divorcing her without obligation. She was very ashamed and felt she had "lost face" among their friends, at the school, and in the community at large. In response, in a fit of anger, Meilin took her daughter and flew back to Taiwan. Tim, fearing for his child, filed a police report claiming "abandonment and child abduction." Meilin returned to the couple's home a few days later, ready to resume their married life. When she learned of the police report she was shocked with disbelief and shaking with rage. In tears, she exclaimed, "How could he do such a thing to his own wife!"

Failure to understand the cultural milieu from which an individual comes can, and often does, lead to incorrect assumptions and conclusions that disrupt and may sometimes permanently damage a marriage.

Incompatibility Between Two Cultures

When two people from different cultures marry, the two "cultures" coexist, side by side, under the same roof. Some cultural norms or beliefs held by the two partners may be incompatible and in conflict.

Some examples may be found in the observance of cultural rituals—wedding ceremonies, for instance—in questions such as where the wedding should take place and who should host and pay for the wedding reception and honeymoon. In American culture, it is the custom for the wedding to take place in the bride's hometown and for the bride's family to finance and host the reception. In Asian culture, the wedding normally takes place in the groom's hometown, and it is planned and financed by the groom's family.

After the marriage, other culturally loaded issues may follow, such as where the couple should live, what names the children should be given, what food should be served, how the children should be raised, what culture(s) the children should identify with, and how much privacy the couple should expect to receive from their extended families. The case of Mary and Kalani demonstrates incompatible views on how children should behave at the dinner table—one spouse feeling they should be allowed to talk, and the other feeling that they should not. Maria and Andy differed in their perceptions and interpretations of who should sit next to the husband in the front seat of the car—the wife, as his mate, or his sister, a guest, to give her a better view.

Different Concepts of Family Boundaries and Obligations

Family structure and dynamics vary in different cultures (Tseng and Hsu 1991). These differences can be, and often are, a source of conflict and problems for intermarried couples (Ratliff et al. 1978). For example, in some cultures, the basic family unit includes only the nuclear family, whereas in others the family unit includes the entire extended family. Boundaries with families of origin and obligations to members of extended families also differ. Mary and Kalani, as well as Maria and Andy, had problems in defining family boundaries and the obligations that go with them.

The following case illustrates how different boundaries and role expectations may cause strains in a marriage:

> Sera, a young mother of Korean background, complained that her German mother-in-law, Helga, traveled often instead of staying home and helping to baby-sit her grandchildren, as a mother-in-law should do. From Sera's cultural perspective, Helga was acting "selfishly" and failing to fulfill the role of a grandmother. Helga, on the other hand, believed that a mother-in-law must respect the independence of the couple and be "careful not to make a pest [of herself] by being underfoot all the time." By traveling often and visiting her grandchildren only occasionally, Helga felt she was ensuring a good relationship with her daughter-in-law.

Conflicts Over Role Division Between Spouses

Perhaps a classic source of problems for intercultural couples is the expected roles and duties assigned to each sex. The lack of common socially ascribed role divisions can cause confusion and conflict. Who is supposed to cook, clean, prepare the bed for a guest, arrange the social schedule, or speak in public on behalf of the couple? Different or unclear expectations on these and other matters are potential areas of conflict. In the case of intramarried couples, these issues are relatively easier to resolve, because the couples share basic, common assumptions. They merely need to adjust their personal styles, on the basis of clearly acknowledged common ground. For interculturally married couples, the so-called common ground is not there or is unclear. The partners need to start from scratch and reach some point of mutual agreement and acceptance—a process that takes special effort and time.

Different Child-Rearing Practices

When the intercultural couple have children, they face another challenge, because different cultures have different methods of and values concerning child rearing. There are issues of how to discipline children, including the means and levels of discipline; how to select and teach the children their primary and second languages; and how to resolve issues regarding the children's ethnic identity (Gibbs 1987). Each of these issues may become a battleground. The identity problems and social adjustment of the children of intermarriages are complex and deserve serious attention (de Snyder and Padilla 1982).

Problems Arising From Community Reaction Toward Intermarriage

The life of any unit, whether it is a couple or a family, is not entirely determined by the individuals participating in it. Life is significantly impacted by an individual's family of origin, extended families, friends, colleagues, the media, government, and other institutions. This impact may be even greater if the couple is interracial. Treatment by relatives, friends, neighbors, and the community is often a crucial factor that affects the marriage itself (Kouri and Lasswell 1993). Andy and Maria (in the case described earlier in this chapter) chose to stay in Hawaii for a simple reason—the multiethnic society of Hawaii accepted the interracially married couple as within the norm and would relate to their future racially mixed children as "local."

In many parts of the world, however, the interracial couple may be substantially disadvantaged. They may be stared at in the street and have difficulty socializing with neighbors, and their children might be teased by schoolmates. One or both will be a minority and may have difficulty obtaining satisfactory employment. Thus, the living environment as a whole, based on people's attitudes toward culture, ethnicity, and race, may have substantial impact, positively or negatively, on the intermarried spouses.

One must strive to avoid generalizations, however, because each case differs in terms of personal factors, the degree of diversity between the cultures involved, differences in physical attributes, reactions of the families on both sides, and, finally, the gender-matching of the ethnic backgrounds. Atkeson (1970), for instance, pointed out that an American husband and a Filipino wife have a better time adjusting than a Filipino husband and an American wife. The cultural definitions and expectations of sex roles, coupled with the ethnic background of the husband and wife, create different outcomes of adjustment. Naturally, the level of adjustment also correlates with the place of residence after marriage. Therefore, each couple's situation must be assessed and understood on a case-by-case basis.

Therapy With Intermarried Couples

Even though therapy for the intermarried couple follows the rules that govern couples' therapy in general, the unique difficulties and challenges that have been described deserve special consideration.

Being Sensitive to the Cultural Perceptions of Therapy Held by Each Partner

Even before formal sessions are started, the therapist needs to be sensitive to the cultural perceptions of therapy held by the couple. People from different cultures may approach therapy with different attitudes and expectations. These differences may interfere with the process and outcome of therapy and need to be addressed at the outset. This is well illustrated in the case of Mary and Kalani, described earlier in this chapter. With his cultural background, Kalani felt that "domestic" problems ought to be resolved among family members themselves and that counseling with a stranger outside of the family was an intrusion into his power as the head of the household. However, Kalani's wife, Mary, felt differently. Indeed, in the initial sessions, Kalani behaved passively and uncooperatively, whereas Mary was active and enthusiastic.

The therapist, if unaware of such cultural differences, could easily be misled and, without knowing it, establish a closer alliance with one of the spouses and alienate the other. Such inequality in alliances may further split the couple and make therapy even more problematic. In this situation, the therapist needs to ameliorate the one spouse's resistance and sense of losing face by respecting his or her position and listening to his or her point of view before supporting and empathizing with the other. Such an approach can be paired with the technique of using culture to reframe the problem. For example, in the case of Mary and Kalani, the therapist could say, "Mary, I know you feel angry and hurt by Kalani's behavior, but Kalani, because of his background and life experiences, must have his reasons. Let's give him a chance to tell us his point of view."

Closely associated with this matter is the influence of different cultural perceptions of authority figures on how the partners may relate to the therapist. For instance, one spouse may come from a culture that is authoritarian and may even view therapy as a form of penalty. In such a case, the individual will wait to be told by the therapist what is wrong and what to do about it. The other spouse may come from a more democratic culture and may see the therapist as an ally, an equal. This individual will commonly relate to the therapist with ease and trust. Knowledge of the cultural background of the partners will help the therapist to recognize and deal with such discrepancies between the ways each partner relates to the therapist.

Considering Ethnic Matching and Therapeutic Neutrality

Establishing good rapport with both partners and avoiding taking sides are crucial from the very beginning of the marital therapy sessions to avoid potential problems and future complications (Hsu 1977). Either partner of a mixed relationship may use the ethnicity of the therapist to threaten the therapist's impartiality by asserting a closer ethnic tie than that with the partner or, conversely, by resisting the therapy more because of greater ethnic distance.

Although outcome studies of individual therapy suggest that the ethnicity or culture of the therapist is not as important as his or her general clinical competence, it is as yet unclear how ethnic matching with the therapist may affect the outcome of therapy with intermarried couples. However, it is clear that the complexities of identification and alienation due to ethnicity, race, or faith need to be monitored and dealt with carefully. Cultural similarity or difference between the therapist and the individuals in the couple is a two-edged sword that can be destructive when unmonitored but very effective when used correctly in therapy.

If the therapist is of the same cultural background as one of the partners, the therapist can use that similarity to provide support and understanding of particular concepts and behaviors, to challenge particular beliefs or customs, or to supplement the positive aspect of a seemingly negative cultural trait or behavior. If the therapist's culture is different from that of one or both partners, this lack of similarity can also be used in therapy. Intense conflicts and emotions can be diffused by soliciting the couple's help in educating the therapist about the one partner's culture and his or her particular situation. Such a request brings the couple together as a team and thereby changes their hostile, opposing positions.

Emphasizing Positive Forces and Common Ground in the Marriage

Regardless of the nature of the problems that exist in the marriage, there must be something good about the partners and the relationship. After all, they did marry, and they agreed to come to therapy to work on their relationship. It is important, despite their problems and cultural differences, to bring out the positive aspects of the relationship. These aspects may include love, care, kids, stability, companionship, sex, and achievement (Jeter 1982). It is also useful to remind the couple that they were once determined to be together and had the strength to accomplish this against all odds. They should be reminded of the difficulties they have faced or knew they might face when deciding to marry. That same resolve and determination can be used to confront and solve their current conflicts and problems. When a couple are in crisis, suffering from many differences and facing negative issues, they need to realize and appreciate the positive aspects in their relationship.

For example, in the case of Mary and Kalani, described earlier, Kalani was reminded of his experience with different cultures during the war and his ability to adapt to them. He was urged to apply this cultural flexibility to adapt to the cultural needs of his wife and daughters. It was pointed out to Mary that Kalani's loyalty to his family of origin also indicated his loyalty to his own nuclear family—that he was a "family man." Mary agreed and pointed out that this aspect of her husband was one that had attracted her to him when they first met.

Promoting Cultural Knowledge, Understanding, and Skills

One of the major problems encountered by intermarried couples is the lack of understanding and appreciation of each other's culture. Specifically, people are unaware that their contrasting viewpoints and behaviors are often based on their different cultural upbringings rather than some problem in the relationship or with the individuals.

It is important for a couple to be able to communicate their complex personal thoughts and deep feelings. Misunderstandings are likely when there is a failure to appreciate the different cultural aspects present in each of the individuals. This lack of appreciation of the other's cultural values is especially exacerbated when the couple do not speak the same language. The language deficiency may also interfere with their social life. Improving the language of one or both spouses may need to be stressed and encouraged.

The therapist needs to help the couple be curious about each other's culture in order to discover, discuss, and understand their differences in beliefs, values, concepts, expectations, and attitudes about many things. The couple must appreciate how such differences affect their interaction and can cause conflict. Openly discussing these matters can help the couple be conscious of and attuned to the cultural differences between them. Often this alone can result in a greatly improved relationship. Once the couple are attuned to each other's cultural aspects, they should be further encouraged to accept and appreciate the positive attributes of each other's culture and to be proud to partake in it as well. The following case illustrates the importance of promoting cultural understanding:

> Toshi, originally from Japan, came to the United States to pursue postgraduate training. He spoke English reasonably well. After his marriage to Nancy, a third-generation American, they started to have problems in communication. Nancy was frustrated that Toshi seldom shared with her what happened at work and no longer praised her or expressed his love for her. Toshi said that he had never seen his own father talk to his mother about work, since work is considered a man's business. He also felt that Nancy should know of his love for her and not need to be told. He felt that he did not need to thank Nancy or praise her, since he regarded such comments as only applying to an "outsider" and not to members of one's own family. After much explanation and encouragement, Toshi was willing to change his behavior, since he now understood Nancy's view and expectations.

Clarifying Cultural Influences Versus Personal Factors

It is common for a person to interpret a spouse's perceived negative behavior as a personal attack. This often generates a great deal of anger and resentment, contributing to conflicts and frustrations. When the couple can view the perceived negative behavior in an intercultural context, they no longer view the behavior as a personal attack, but rather as an expression of the individual's cultural beliefs.

However, it is as common to "culturalize" as to "personalize" the problem. A person may identify his or her partner's ethnicity or culture as the cause of the behavior and thereby fail to look into personal and relationship issues. Perceiving personal or relationship problems as solely cultural can interfere with effective communication and delay resolution of the real conflict.

A task for the therapist is to be a "cultural referee," helping the couple clarify which behaviors are rooted in culture, and which are better seen as manifestations of the person or the relationship. On the other hand, when it is suitable to do so, the therapist may use culture as a way to "reframe" the cause of conflict in order to reduce anger and resentment and to promote good feelings. In such a case, stereotyping can actually be helpful. For example, telling a wife who is angry at her husband for not showing affection and not being available, "Toshi is a typical Japanese husband," is using the ethnic stereotype of Japanese being hard-working but shy in expressing emotions. However, the therapist needs to avoid the risk that such a statement may be used as an excuse for not changing toward better ways of relating. In general, the statement is better followed by the request that Toshi be more expressive and available in spite of his ethnic background.

Promoting Flexibility and Appreciation of Differences

It is useful for the therapist to stress that there is no right or wrong between various cultures, only differences. The therapist can help the couple to understand not only that their differences are perfectly acceptable but also that these differences can have a positive impact on the relationship. The therapist needs to function as a cultural broker both to encourage the couple in their appreciation of and adaptation to their cultures and to liberate them from rigid cultural restraints. The couple can find a modified middle path that suits both cultures, or at least find a path that does not conflict with either culture. A new, more liberated family tradition can be formed. The couple can, alternatively or in addition, practice customs of both cultures at different times and on separate occasions (Tseng 1977).

The therapist can help the couple develop concrete steps to adjust to each other's culture, such as taking language lessons, participating in culture programs or activities, or allowing "cultural holidays." Each spouse is allowed to have a cultural holiday, or cultural regression, during which that spouse is encouraged to practice the rites, rituals, activities, behaviors, and traditions of his or her culture of origin.

The therapy will benefit when the advantages of multiculturalism in a family are emphasized: differences do not always create conflict; they can also generate broader perspectives, greater knowledge, and multiple ways to enjoy life, to deal with problems, and to meet challenges. Instead of assigning negative traits to each partner's respective culture, the couple can attribute positive qualities to their different cultural values and patterns and learn to appreciate and enjoy the differences.

Avoiding Therapeutic Approaches That May Be Too Culture-Specific

Certain time-honored approaches in couples therapy may be more, if not solely, suitable for Euro-American couples and should be avoided or used with great caution when treating intermarried couples.

Role playing, for example, can facilitate communication and expression of emotion and provide opportunities for intervention in the session. For Americans or Europeans who value open communication and public sharing of affection and who have little fear of confrontation, role playing is an effective therapeutic tool. This is usually not the case for individuals of other cultures. For example, Asians traditionally view expressions of emotions in public, especially negative emotions, as an indication of having lost one's self-control. For these individuals, open confrontation with each other in the presence of the therapist exposes "family ugliness" to an "outsider," a betrayal in the worst form. Additionally, "acting" used to be considered a profession of rather low social status; therefore, no Asian man with self-respect would role-play without great reluctance. Asking a Japanese husband to play an assigned role can be interpreted as an insult to the man.

Paradoxical intention, with its effectiveness resting as it does on the rebelliousness of the client, can be harmful if one spouse comes from a culture that encourages one to listen and obey authority. For example, suggesting divorce to a couple with chronic conflict of the "can't live with and can't live without" type may not obtain the expected response: the couple's determination to improve the relationship in order to show that the therapist is wrong. On the contrary, the couple may be confused or even angry at the therapist for "instructing" them to divorce each other, which may be unacceptable by their cultures.

Conclusion

All couples have difficulties in adapting to each other. Variations in racial, ethnic, or cultural background might lead to additional difficulties and challenges to the usual challenges faced in marriage. Marital problems may derive from many sources, such as incompatibility of personalities, unsound motivations, different philosophies about life, different expectations of marriage and the role of the spouse, and so on. For intermarried couples, whose difficulties also include different culture-rooted beliefs and traditions, the challenge of therapy is all the greater for everyone involved.

The principles and strategies used in therapy with intermarried couples are not fundamentally different from those used with ordinary (intramarried) couples. There is no unique mode of treating intermarried couples; however, certain issues definitely need more attention and special consideration. In these cases, the therapist must also promote cultural curiosity, knowledge, and understanding and increased tolerance of the other's culture. This can be achieved by encouraging appreciation, flexibility of interpretation, the practice of multiculturalism in the family, and establishment of a modernized, hybrid, new family tradition.

Finally, it needs to be emphasized that intermarriage itself should not be conceptualized as a marriage with inherited problems and difficulties in adjustment. With the mutual adjustment of both spouses, the marriage can be very successful (Tseng 1977). Such adjustment is more likely when the spouses have flexible personalities, are open-minded, are curious, appreciate innovative experiences, are capable of adapting to various situations, and are eager to learn about their partners. In a sense, couples who intermarry against possible resistance and succeed in overcoming problems demonstrate higher levels of commitment to each other and higher levels of coping than do other couples.

References

Atkeson P: Building communication in intercultural marriage. Psychiatry 33:396–408, 1970

Cohen N: Same or different? A problem in identity in cross-cultural marriages. Journal of Family Therapy 4:177–199, 1982

Davidson JR: Theories about Black-White interracial marriage: a clinical perspective. Journal of Multicultural Counseling and Development 20:150–157, 1992

Gibbs JT: Identity and marginality: issues in the treatment of biracial adolescents. Am J Orthopsychiatry 57:265–278, 1987

Hsu J: Counseling for intercultural marriage, in Adjustment in Intercultural Marriage. Edited by Tseng WS, McDermott JF Jr, Maretzki TW. Honolulu, Department of Psychiatry, University of Hawaii, 1977, pp 121-132

Jeter K: Analytic essay: intercultural and interracial marriage. Marriage and Family Review 5:105–111, 1982

Kitano HH, Yeung WT, Chai L, et al: Asian-American interracial marriage. Journal of Marriage and the Family 46:179–190, 1984

Kouri KM, Lasswell M: Black-white marriages: social change and intergenerational mobility. Marriage and Family Review 19:241–255, 1993

Ratliff BW, Moon HF, Bonacci GA: Intercultural marriage: the Korean-American experience. Social Casework 59:221–226, 1978

de Snyder SN, Padilla AM: Interethnic marriages of Mexican Americans after nearly two decades (Spanish Speaking Mental Health Research Center Occasional Papers 15). Los Angeles, Spanish Speaking Mental Health Research Center, University of California at Los Angeles, 1982

Solsberry PW: Interracial couples in the United States of America: implications for mental health counseling. Journal of Mental Health Counseling 16:304–317, 1994

Tseng WS: Adjustment in intercultural marriage, in Adjustment in Intercultural Marriage. Edited by Tseng WS, McDermott JF Jr, Maretzki TW. Honolulu, Department of Psychiatry, University of Hawaii, 1977, pp 93–103

Tseng WS, Hsu J: Culture and Family: Problems and Therapy. New York, Haworth Press, 1991

CHAPTER 16

Group Therapy With Multiethnic Members

Leslie Ann Matsukawa, M.D.

Cultural factors influence how a person relates to others and, therefore, interactions with members of a group and with the leader of the group. In a multiethnic society, it is natural for therapy groups to be composed of members with widely varying backgrounds and widely varying values, beliefs, and attitudes. Thus, conducting culturally relevant and effective group therapy with multiethnic members is an exciting clinical challenge to the contemporary group therapist.

Culture and Group Therapy: Literature Review

Ethnically Homogeneous Groups

Most of the existing literature on ethnic and cultural aspects of group psychotherapy deals with homogeneous groups of ethnic minorities in the United States. The research has focused on variations of dynamics and techniques in conducting therapy with groups whose members are composed of a particular ethnic background.

Hispanic Groups

Hynes and Werbin (1977) co-led a group of Hispanic women, combining supportive, ventilatory, and problem-solving approaches with relaxation techniques. As part of the supportive and flexible approach, transportation to and from the sessions and rotating child care were provided to the members.

Olarte and Masnik (1985) pointed out modifications of technique needed to foster comfort and participation in psychotherapy groups for Hispanic persons at a mental health clinic in New York City. Various topics were introduced at the beginning of each session for discussion in go-arounds, including family conflicts, child rearing, and drug and alcohol problems. Members did not talk about their personal experiences with these things, but they did present what they knew about such matters. This lack of disclosure was not challenged by the therapist, who understood that to talk directly at the onset about one's intimate problems would be very guilt-inspiring, akin to a confession. Psychoeducation by the therapist allowed the group members to self-reveal gradually, since it was taught that talking about one's problems was the route to understanding how to solve them. Another useful technical modification was the use of traditional music, celebrations, and foods to promote cohesion and comfort in the group.

Delgado (1983), in describing the values shared by Hispanic peoples, stressed the importance of mobilizing Hispanic group members' support systems, including the extended family, social clubs, church, and so forth. The fostering of a personal, friendly relationship through visits to meet family members helped the therapist form a strong therapeutic alliance with the group members.

Other Ethnic Minority Groups

Wolman (1970) worked with a group of Navajo people, most of whom were bilingual and some of whom spoke no English. He modeled cohesiveness by urging the bilingual member who was solely speaking English in the group to translate for the non–English speaking members.

Kinzie et al. (1988) discussed meeting concrete needs and providing socialization experiences via traditional activities, such as cooking, handicrafts, and music, in groups of Indo-Chinese refugees.

Davis (1984), in working with groups of African Americans, urged looking for the roots of behavior both within the individual and within the social milieu. From this process would flow interventions with support systems outside of the group that were necessary for the well-being of the group members.

C. P. Chen (1995) discussed modifications of technique that were useful in working with Chinese groups in Canada. He noted that the group members tended to expect the therapist to maintain the image of an authority figure, to educate the members, and to provide structure for the group process.

Groups in Other Countries

Group psychotherapy in Japan was discussed by Yamaguchi (1986), who stressed the family-like atmosphere of groups, in which the members pull together to provide one another with support and solutions. He suggested that the value of "groupism," or mutuality, may tend to make the group therapy situation more comfortable than individual therapy for many Japanese people.

C. C. Chen (1972) described group experiences with Chinese patients in Taiwan, which were characterized by discussion of preselected topics in a structured manner for psychoeducational purposes.

In Russia, Gilbert and Shiryaev (1992) reported that, although psychoanalysis had been considered ideologically unacceptable prior to glasnost, group therapy has been popular and widely practiced. They pointed out that Russia, especially during the years of Soviet domination, has traditionally been a group-oriented society, and forces of social influence present in therapy groups could exert a powerful effect on group members.

Ethnically Heterogeneous Groups

The workings of an ethnically/racially and culturally diverse psychotherapy group are fascinating and are now being recognized for their great potential in changing the attitudes and behavior of its members. Warriner (1978) warned about the danger of thinking of race as the only, or the most important, distinguishing characteristic of individuals in the group, and suggested techniques for promoting cohesion in a diverse, transcultural group.

Vasquez and Han (1995) described the therapeutic factors of validation, empowerment, mutuality, and self-empathy in multicultural groups. Race affects the dynamics of multiethnic groups and must be openly explored, with a working-through of feelings about race and culture, for such groups to work effectively (Davis 1984; White 1994).

Tsui and Schultz (1988) illustrated defensive maneuvers that arise in ethnically heterogeneous groups. They discussed how these maneuvers could sabotage the group process, unless they are recognized and their possible cultural origins are understood. From experiences with clinical groups that included African Americans clients, Davis (1984) feels that interracial groups succeed if the therapist is able to convey to the clients that he or she understands their sociocultural position as well as their personal issues.

Cultural Values Influencing Group Dynamics

People with different ethnic and cultural backgrounds bring varied and contrasting values, particularly in regard to interpersonal relations, into the social microcosm of a psychotherapy group. Ethnically derived values, involving the issues of mutuality versus individualism, social hierarchy, and ethnic identification, influence the way members interact with others in the group.

Members' expectations and goals in a multiethnic group vary widely according to what each individual deems as important in his or her relationships. These value-driven expectations will significantly influence the dynamics of the therapy group. In order to be effective, the group leader must take into consideration these differing ethnically derived values and understand their effect on the dynamics of the group. This understanding will lead to certain modifications of technique, necessary to promote therapeutic change in multiethnic psychotherapy group members.

Mutuality Versus Individualism

The status of the self in regard to the other affects how an individual relates to other group members. The self is valued on a continuum of individualism versus mutuality. Where one sees oneself on this continuum helps determine the psychological boundaries between the self and any group, including a family unit. Many Asian cultures view the self as intimately connected with the group (Chu and Sue 1984; Tsui and Schultz 1988). For instance, many Japanese people are group-minded and seek to promote the good of the group, even at personal expense. The old saying goes, "If the nail is sticking up, you pound it back down." The personal characteristic of *enryo,* or holding back or restraint, is highly valued; it can be seen in the group setting, where, instead of asserting himself or herself and making his or her opinions known, the Japanese member may sit back and let others take the lead. One hesitates to call attention to oneself directly, because this would take time and attention away from others and be considered "showing off."

Another manifestation of the self as highly connected to the other is implicit in the view held by many Asian families that an illness or problem of one of the family members is the responsibility of the entire family because it reflects on the rest of the family (Tsui and Schultz 1985).

A second-generation Japanese American man was in a therapy group made up of parents of drug- and alcohol-dependent adult children. The ethnic composition of the group was Japanese, Chinese, Portuguese, and Caucasian. In the first session, he stated softly, hanging his head, "I don't know how he came out like this," and went on to talk about his son's stealing from the family to pay for drugs, looking increasingly ashamed as he proceeded. The other members, including the other Japanese Americans, reassured him with statements such as, "Oh, it's not your fault; you shouldn't blame yourself," "My daughter stole from us, too," "Yeah, you know, you try to raise them right but they still go to the drugs." The cotherapists, a fourth-generation Japanese American woman and a Portuguese and Hawaiian American woman, jointly reiterated what a pervasive problem drug and alcohol abuse is, pointing out how no families are untouched. The Japanese American man then replied, "But it was my fault." He poured out his regrets over having been too focused on his work and neglecting his family, having been too harsh a disciplinarian, and not having understood what his son needed from him emotionally.

It is of utmost importance in a multiethnic psychotherapy group to create an environment in which group members feel safe to reveal cultural values and their personal meaning. Tsui and Schultz (1985) explained the way an illness (or mental illness) becomes a family stigma and the social responsibility of the family. Particularly with mental illness, there can be a fear that the family will be blamed should the ill family member do something shameful. The Japanese American man's initial statement, "I don't know how he came out like this," masked a deep sense of responsibility and regret over not having been able to connect with his son. He felt very ashamed and guilty over his son's drug use.

The group members' response to the shame on this member's face was to try to relieve him of the guilt, pointing out commonalities in their situations with their children. The cotherapists promoted the safety he felt by re-emphasizing the universality of what he was experiencing with his son. This therapeutic modification came out of the recognition that, partly because of his ethnic background, he may have been taking on the blame for his son's illness. Any questioning of him on his relationship with his son or on his initial statement of disavowal would have increased his shame. Once he saw that he was not going to be blamed by the others, he felt safe to reveal his feelings of immense guilt. By the end of the session, in which he was educated about the nature of addictions and gained support from the group, he was greatly relieved, and joked, "So I guess it wasn't entirely my fault." Being thus relieved, he was able to go home and confront his son about his behavior and then set limits on him, with the support of the group.

Social Role and Hierarchy

The way one looks at role relationships is often culturally determined. There is a continuum of cultures in terms of roles and status, from those that are highly stratified to those that are more amorphous. The Filipino value of *amor proprio,* which is manifested as pride in the telling of one's position and status (Ponce 1980), leads to a communication style that may be off-putting in an ethnically mixed psychotherapy group.

> A 40-year-old Filipino American man, born in the Philippines and living in Hawaii for the past 20 years, had lost his job due to a work-related injury. For the first four sessions of a time-limited, interpersonal group, he brought up how well-to-do he had been—how he had two fancy cars and a very expensive home. After the first few sessions, other members of the group would roll their eyes whenever he began talking in this manner. The group leader called attention to the nonverbal communication and asked the group, consisting of Japanese, Filipino, and Caucasian members, what was going on. Complete silence ensued. Invited by the therapist to say what he thought might be going on, the Filipino man spoke up after a few more moments of silence in the group and stated, "I say too much about how great a man I was. It's because I have nothing now, I have to remind myself what I had before."

In Filipino societies, which have a very strict hierarchical social alignment, by making oneself and one's accomplishments known to others, one quickly establishes a place in the milieu (Ponce 1980). The other members of this multi-ethnic group did not understand that this was the Filipino man's accustomed way of entering into a group. The group leader explained the concept of *amor proprio,* with input by the Filipino members. This explanation of a culturally based style of presenting oneself, along with the Filipino-American man's realization that he was alienating other people, helped the other members empathize with the man and tolerate his self-laudatory speech, and allowed them to accept what he in turn had to offer, which was a considerable amount of understanding and supportive camaraderie.

The therapeutic modification needed in this multiethnic group situation would be for the therapist to help a person explain to the other members the particular values motivating his behavior (Tsui and Schultz 1988). Instead of probing the other members about the silence and eliciting from someone the painfully obvious reason for the eye rolling, which would have shamed the Filipino member, the therapist invited the member to explain his need to promote himself. The therapist had observed that the member was seeing the eye-rolling of the others and appeared to shrink in his seat when this occurred. By putting the nonverbal response toward him on the table, and asking the Filipino member to give his response to it, the therapist helped the member convey to the others his own self-awareness and embarrassment. This led to a heightening of empathy toward him by the others and a subsequent decrease in his self-aggrandizement.

Ethnic Identity

Comas-Diaz and Jacobsen (1987) and Gehrie (1979) have written about the importance of culture and ethnicity in the development of a stable sense of self. The multiethnic group experience brings to the fore and accentuates one's feelings about race and ethnicity (White 1994). Conflicts about one's attachments to one's ethnic group often emerge early in the course of the group.

> A 30-year-old Chinese woman who immigrated from Taiwan had severe, recurrent depressive episodes and could not work. She lived with her parents and felt very ashamed about relying on them for support. In the second session of a multiethnic interpersonal group therapy, she stated, "There is a Chinese saying: 'Your father gives you clothes. Your mother gives you food.' Some of my parents' friends have said that to them. It makes me feel very bad."

> A 40-year-old woman of Guatemalan Mexican descent, born in Hawaii to immigrant parents, spoke of her experiences in high school and how she was thought to be part-Hawaiian and part-Chinese because of her looks. "People would come up and say, 'Eh, what you? You look *local,* but you get one funny accent.' I would just tell them I had a speech impediment."

> A woman of Hawaiian and Chinese descent would shift in her primary ethnic identity, depending on her moods and situations in the multiethnic group therapy. When she was depressed, she identified with the harsh Chinese grandmother who had raised her from age 6 years, who spoke perfect English. At such times, the patient would sit silently through much of the session, except for occasional sharp criticisms of the spouses that other members were talking about or of the cotherapists, delivered in perfect English. When she was hypomanic, she identified with the easygoing, loving, but ineffectual Hawaiian father, who, unable to handle his grief, left her after her mother died. During these times, she would speak pidgin English and would make light of members' concerns in the group.

According to White (1994), a multiethnic group stimulates more talking about race/ethnicity, both one's own and that of others. She goes on to say that one's ethnic identity is affected by the stereotypes and prejudices that abound about particular ethnic groups. In the first case described above, involving the Chinese woman from Taiwan, her sense of identity as a use-less, helpless woman was the result of not only her illness but the attitude toward females in the society from which she came. Gehrie (1979) noted that one's culture becomes a source of either pride or disappointment, de-pending on the ability of one's parents to pass on cultural ideals. This wom-an's parents were unempathetic and rigid in their expectations of her, and this led her to be extremely sensitive to what her culture demanded and what she was failing to live up to. She could not meet her cultural ideal, and her need for belonging left her depressed and empty. A similar dynamic occurred in the third case described above, regarding the woman of Hawaiian and Chi-nese descent who had a shifting, unstable sense of ethnic self. In the second case, the woman with the Hispanic accent, who denied her ethnic back-ground, had grown up in an atmosphere of racial intolerance, in which one would get beaten up if one were "different." This led to her internalization of a devalued and powerless ethnic identity.

The therapeutic modification needed in multiethnic group therapy with members such as these is the promotion of empowerment and self-empathy (Vasquez and Han 1995). Members were urged by other members and co-therapists of other ethnicities to abandon their devalued and idealized ste-reotypes of what was expected of them, and their strengths and possible new roles were encouraged. This led to an increase in self-esteem. An example of this process was an interaction between a Chinese woman from Taiwan and a woman recently emigrated from Germany who were in the same group for therapy. The Chinese woman spoke of how embarrassed she was when she was out with a friend and found herself unable to think of anything to talk about. After a few moments of silence, the German woman ventured, "Did you feel like you had to talk? Maybe it's something cultural, but in my coun-try, it is a great compliment if you can just sit with a friend, without needing to talk. It shows how close you are." The therapist then encouraged the Chi-nese woman to think of what was just said to her, "So, like she says, maybe you don't have to feel pressured to think up conversation." The following session, the Chinese woman thanked the German woman for the suggestion, saying that it made her feel good and that she even answered a phone call from one of her friends, despite fearing she would not know what to talk about.

Dynamics Specific to Multiethnic Psychotherapy Groups

Among the dynamic processes often seen in multiethnic psychotherapy groups, four specific ones will be discussed here: symbolism and nonverbal communication, cultural transference, cultural countertransference, and ethnic prejudice.

Symbolism and Nonverbal Communication

A Japanese American woman in her 50s, who had problems with panic attacks and depression, participated in a time-limited, multiethnic psychotherapy group. The other members of the group were of Irish German, Chinese Hawaiian, Polish, Chinese, and Portuguese American backgrounds. The cotherapists, both women, were of Japanese-Okinawan American and Italian-Irish American descent. The Japanese American woman's self-esteem was very low, and she talked about sensing that her father had felt that she was "good for nothing" when she was growing up, because of her numerous health problems and physical weakness. At the start of the session after she spoke of this, she opened her bag and brought out her handiwork: beaded jewelry and crocheted baby clothes she had made. She did this without a word. The group, led by the cotherapists, praised her for her talent. The cotherapists then thanked her for showing the group this creative part of herself.

Chu and Sue (1984), Knobel (1990) and Morsbach (1973) emphasize the importance of *symbolic and nonverbal communication* in different ethnic and cultural groups. Because of the cultural inhibition of the direct verbal expression of feelings and thoughts in certain Asian group members, symbolic gestures, such as the sharing of food or the bringing of gifts, may help these members express affiliation and belonging (Chu and Sue 1984). *Omoiyari*, a personal attribute valued by the Japanese, is defined as the ability to be highly sensitive to the feelings and desires of others, without them having to tell you directly what they want (Sugiyama-Lebra 1976). One is to help others satisfy their wishes, without being told what they are. This valued aspect of interpersonal relations leads to a communication style and self-expression that are indirect, relying heavily on symbolism and nonverbal signals (Tamura and Lau 1992). Morsbach (1973) illustrates common nonverbal aspects of communication in Japan, such as facial expressions, yawning, eye contact, voice tones, and sounds such as grunting.

The Japanese American woman who brought in her handiwork, feeling so devalued and unsure of herself, took a risk by bringing in the things she had made as a representation of her abilities. It was early in the course of a time-limited group. Being quite traditional in her values, she was stepping out a bit from the *enryo*, or restraint, and was able to show her talent, as long as she did not have to use her words. She symbolically showed an important part of herself in a way that led to a deepening of the trust and cohesion of the group. The modification in therapeutic approach was to allow her to *symbolically* present herself, without questioning, taking into account her cultural prohibition against verbal self-aggrandizement. The "acting in" was not interpreted because the cotherapists realized that her nonverbal communication about herself was quite moving and effective. Her talent was appreciated by the group, and her self-esteem rose. She went on to start her own small business, selling her handicrafts.

Flexibility and empathy are required of the group therapist, who must be willing to recognize and explore the nonverbal communication (Knobel 1990). The therapist must be willing to model nonverbal communication, when appropriate and useful. With such varied and contrasting styles and levels of verbal communicativeness in a multiethnic group, it is interesting to observe how nonverbal communication sometimes becomes a more important and attended-to method of interrelating. Just as the initially less verbal members start to experiment with expressing more of their feelings, because of the modeling of verbal expression by other members and the leader in a safe atmosphere, the more verbal members start picking up on and using nonverbal signals. I have observed that affirmative head nodding and smiling when members recognize universally shared experiences are more evident in a multiethnic psychotherapy group than in a group more homogeneous for ethnicity, especially when these responses are modeled by the leader. The interest in and importance attached to facial expression were underscored for the author, a Japanese-Okinawan American, by a comment written by one of the members of a multiethnic group that she co-led. At the end of a session, the group members each were asked to write down the single thing that they felt was most helpful in the session. A Hawaiian-Filipino-Chinese woman wrote, "Watching my doctor's expression. With interest and understanding. It's an enlightenment."

In addition to modeling nonverbal communication, the therapist should be willing to intervene and help members explain their message when a nonverbal signal they are giving is misinterpreted. At times, Japanese people may smile when they are feeling uncomfortable, upset, sad, or angry (Morsbach 1973). Such a culturally influenced nonverbal signal could easily be misinterpreted by members of other ethnicities.

When a Portuguese American woman was talking about fighting with her husband, a Japanese American woman seated opposite her was smiling uncomfortably. The Portuguese American woman said angrily, "It's not funny!" The Japanese American woman appeared shocked but kept smiling. After a few moments of silence, the therapist intervened, "I wonder if you are upset because she is smiling?" addressing the Portuguese American woman. Then, turning to the Japanese American woman, "Maybe you could explain to her what is making you smile." The Japanese American woman replied, "Habit, I guess. I smile when I'm feeling bad for someone." The Portuguese American woman then said, "Oh, sorry, I thought you were making fun of me."

As Morsbach (1973) explained, smiling at times of discomfort may help the Japanese summon inner reserves and bear up under the strain of the situation. In the case above, it was also a way that the Japanese American member showed her empathy. The therapeutic modification required that the therapist observe and point out the nonverbal communication as the source of discomfort to the Portuguese American woman and then ask the sender of the nonverbal communication to put it into words, if she could. This opened up a vital discussion of how a person's intentions may be misinterpreted. The need to check out confusing messages with the sender, in order to better understand each other, was emphasized.

Cultural Transference

Cultural transference is defined as the feelings and reactions that a member has toward a therapist of a different ethnic background, based on the past experiences that the member has had with people of the same ethnicity as the therapist's (Ridley 1989). These are automatic negative or positive reactions, simply based on the therapist's ethnicity.

> A Hawaiian-Chinese American woman in her 40s had been raised by her Chinese grandmother in a household of Chinese-German-Irish-English American cousins. In a session that marked the midpoint of a time-limited, multiethnic group psychotherapy, this member announced to the Irish-Italian American cotherapist, "I don't know if you can handle my problems. You remind me of my *haole* [Caucasian] cousins." When asked if she could explain, she talked in length about her cousins, whom she looked upon as "weaker" than she was. She spoke of how they were delicate and reserved, and how she, in contrast, was loud and spoke her mind "local [Hawaii] style," as she put it. Addressing the Irish-Italian American cotherapist, she stated, "They [the cousins] always looked at me like they were shocked, or something. I think I might be too much for you. You might not be able to handle me. Dr. Miyasato, [addressing the other cotherapist, a Japanese-Okinawan American woman], she can handle. She looks tougher."

Ridley (1989) advocates the careful recognition and examination of the cultural transference in order to reveal and resolve the intrapsychic conflicts that may underlie it. The behavior that a member displays toward the therapists in the group may be rooted in the expectations the member has toward them because of the member's past experiences with people of the same ethnicity (ethnicities) as the therapists'. In the vignette above, the member was attributing to the Caucasian therapist the befuddlement and dismay she saw in her Chinese Caucasian cousins' eyes. The member devalued the Caucasian therapist and idealized the Asian cotherapist.

> Instead of interpreting the cultural transference or the splitting, the Irish-Italian American cotherapist made a technical modification by revealing something about herself in relation to the Hawaiian-Chinese American member. She revealed that the look in her eyes of surprise and puzzlement when the member was speaking was the result of her not understanding some of the "local" or pidgin English used by the member at times, but that it was also an expression of wonder and admiration of the woman for being able to speak her mind. Many of the other group members joined in and expressed their admiration and gratitude for the member's straightforward manner. The Irish-Italian American cotherapist went on to say that she would make more of an effort to ask the member to translate the pidgin English when necessary and also to make more of a conscious effort to let the member know what she thought of her. The member then thanked the cotherapist, adding, "I probably jumped to conclusions about you and wasn't giving you a chance." She then started opening up to the previously devalued cotherapist and found that she could be accepted and understood by her. Outside of the group, her defensiveness with members of her family started to decrease, and one by one, her relatives started to approach her, after having been estranged for some years. By the end of the 24-week group, she had reunited with her grandmother and cousins.

So much of the cultural transference is based on "jumping to conclusions," and thinking that one knows what the other person is thinking about them, because of their past experiences with others. The cotherapist's modeling of self-revelation about her feelings toward the member decreased the member's defensiveness and increased the safety in the group for the expression of both negative and positive feelings. The cotherapist gained the members' alliance in helping themselves to be understood.

Cultural Countertransference

Ridley (1989) defines *cultural countertransference* as the reaction of a therapist to a client of a different ethnic group, based on past reactions to others of that ethnic group. The experience of cultural countertransference is illustrated in the next vignette.

> A time-limited, interpersonal psychotherapy group consisted of people of diverse ethnic, cultural, and racial backgrounds. They all had problems

with depression, anxiety, and difficulties being understood by important people in their lives. In the first session of this group, the African American woman spoke of growing up in Philadelphia and of a traumatic experience of being spit on by a Caucasian teenager. The French American woman downplayed the racism the African American woman was exposed to, stating, "You know how punk kids are; that could've happened to anyone . . . it might not have been just because you're black." The therapist, a Japanese American, felt quite irritated at the French American member, who, she thought, being Caucasian, probably had never experienced racism and was trying to deny its existence. The therapist grunted, "Ungh," expressionless, and remained silent, although she wanted to scold the French American woman for her denial. The African American woman shot fire from her eyes for a second at the French American woman, then replied, evenly, "Let me tell you how black people are treated here . . .," and went on about other episodes of racial discrimination she had had to deal with in her life.

Ticho (1971) explained the phenomenon of cultural stereotyping as it appears in transference and countertransference in cross-cultural psychotherapy. She feels that the particular aspects of the racial stereotype that the patient and the therapist put on each other should be examined, as they are illustrative of the dynamics operating. White (1994) pointed out that by exploring the feelings about another's race that come up in individual and group therapy, the psychodynamic issues underlying them may emerge. Tylim (1982) vividly described countertransference in a group psychotherapy with Hispanic patients, in which he was idealized and, not wanting to burst their bubble, felt overprotective and entirely responsible for their stability.

In the vignette above, the therapist's cultural countertransference was clearly operating on a number of levels. As a member of an ethnic minority herself, she felt hostile to the Caucasian woman for denying an act of racial malice, and she felt overprotective of the African American woman. Luckily, she restrained herself from saying anything while in the midst of a countertransference storm, and the African American woman was able to tell the group more about what she had suffered because of racism. Many of the group members, and the therapist, shook their heads in shared anger over what this woman had experienced, and this helped the African American woman feel understood and validated. Many expressed shock and horror, stating, "I just can't believe what you've gone through," and "I can't believe people could be that cruel!"

The therapist observed that this element of disbelief was consensually validated in the group, and this lessened the anger toward the French American woman for doubting the racist motivation of the spitting. The therapist felt the need to help the group address the denial, stating, "I think that be-cause it's hard to hear about a person being treated so badly because of race, there's a tendency to deny that such a thing could happen." The French American woman took her cue and immediately responded, addressing the African American woman, "Yeah, I'm sorry I was downplaying that kid's behavior. Hearing about it just made me ashamed of my whole family, who tried to teach me that you hate black people. I broke away from that. I couldn't see the sense in it, hating someone because of their skin color." The African American woman acknowledged her apology with a nod. The therapist's own personal anger toward the French American woman dissolved with hearing her need, initially, to deny the existence of racism.

Ethnic Prejudice

Ethnic stereotyping, or the labeling of certain ethnic groups with generalized traits and characteristics, becomes quite evident in a multiethnic psycho-therapy group. It is a mechanism that people use to get their bearings. It is also used to deal with the culture shock of being with strangers who are for-eign and unknown and with whom they are expected to feel comfortable enough to talk. Stereotypes become prejudices when they are hard to modify and when one's interactions, or lack thereof, with another person are based on preconceived feelings and judgments about the person's race, without enough knowledge, understanding, or experience. Prejudice, too, occurs in a multiethnic group, especially in the initial and differentiation stages of a time-limited group. It can result in scapegoating and threatens the cohesive-ness of the group if it is not attended to and worked through.

> A Samoan American woman attended the first two sessions of a multiethnic psychotherapy group, talking mostly about her difficulties disciplining and providing for her five young children. She was absent the following session. An African American woman, Mary, who had six children, commented that the Samoan American woman was probably having problems with her chil-dren, keeping her away from therapy that day. An English-Danish Ameri-can man replied, angrily, looking at the therapist, "If these women have such trouble dealing with their kids, why do they keep having so many? They all end up on welfare." The therapist responded, "Why don't you ask?" Before he could ask, Mary, the African American woman, replied, looking straight at the man, "If you wanna know why I had so many kids, well, I grew up in not such a great area in Chicago, and the building I lived in, my father was the janitor for. Well, I used to help him downstairs with the trash and all, and we would find dead babies, some of them wrapped up, some just thrown away in the alley, like somebody just dropped them out the window to get rid of them. I couldn't have been more than 8 or 9

years old when I remember saying to myself, 'If those were my babies, I would have loved them and fed them, and never would've let anything happen to them.'"

A Samoan American woman was talking about the abusive relationship she had with her ex-husband. She was recounting how he used to demand that she drop everything she was doing and serve him his food the minute he walked in the door. She stated she got fed up with this and yelled at him, "What I look like to you—black?! I ain't a slave." There was complete silence in the room until the African American woman in the group responded, "As you can see, I am black. No, this is not a tan, I'm black. And we weren't no slaves, either. There is no man I would let treat me like that."

During the last session of a time-limited multiethnic psychotherapy group, an Irish-English-Scottish American woman talked about going to a multi-specialty medical clinic and seeing a new surgical resident. "And you should have seen him. It's the first time in all my years down there that I ever got a good-looking doctor. All the rest were Oriental or from Kuka-monga or somewhere, who knows!? They all have accents. No offense, but they're just not my type." A cotherapist and one other member were Asian.

From the very start of a multiethnic therapy group, people must be made to feel that race is a topic that is safe to discuss (Davis 1984). If the topic is ignored or not explored, scapegoating and division along racial lines can occur (Tsui and Schultz 1988). It is my experience that comments about race, one's own and that of the group members, come up frequently and quite early in the course of a multiethnic group. During one particular 12-session, time-limited interpersonal group, race came up in the first five sessions, as did money, religion, and politics. This was quite different from my experience in more racially homogeneous groups, in which the initial sessions are notable for people searching for superficial commonalties and ways to identify with each other. It is almost as if members of multiethnic groups are testing the waters to see if, being so different from each other in race, social background, and values, they will still be safe and accepted.

In the first vignette in this subsection, the stereotyping of "these women with so many kids" led the English-Danish American man to be angry toward racial minority women, who he felt were irresponsible in having so many children. This ethnic prejudice had to be addressed, and the therapist felt hopeful that any one of a number of the minority women in the group would be able to reveal something about herself that would dispel that man's stereotype of her. The African American woman spoke up after the therapist made it clear that the man could find out the answer to his question by asking the group—that it was a safe topic. The question posed to the group after the African American woman spoke was, "How does it make you feel toward Mary, hearing of her experience?" The effect on the group, and this man in particular, was a deepening in understanding of her overprotectiveness of her children and a chipping away at the prejudice.

In the second vignette, the slave comment caused an initial shock and anxiety response in the cotherapists, who looked at each other, wide-eyed, and thought to themselves "Uh-oh!" As in most cases of a racially noxious remark, group members can address the issue if they feel safe enough that the anger and anxiety, and whatever other emotion arises, can be contained and worked through in the group. The African American woman defused the anxiety by making a humorous reference to people's "color-blindness" and casually thrown-about racist remarks. She then asserted herself with the Samoan American woman, saying she would never let a man make her subservient, and then went on to give the woman advice on how to leave him. The Samoan American woman replied, gratefully, "Thanks, sistah, that's good advice." The cotherapists then commented on the way the interaction played out and encouraged discussion about people's reactions to racially offensive remarks and their experiences with handling ethnic prejudice.

In the third vignette, several dynamics were played out, besides the obvious racial stereotyping and ethnic prejudice. There was the Irish-English-Scottish American woman's anger at the therapist for the group's ending, as well as her general dissatisfaction with the medical clinic in which she felt that her physical complaints were not taken seriously. But the pointed "Oriental" reference had to be addressed first. The therapist replied, "But I do take offense [with a very serious affect]. You see, I'm from Kukamonga." The group members laughed, and then the therapist pointed out, "You know, even if you didn't mean to offend, I'm wondering if there is actually something going on behind your comment about 'Orientals,' seeing how Ailin [the Asian member] and I are Asian." The Irish-English-Scottish American woman replied, "Well, there I go again, putting my big foot in my mouth. I really didn't mean anything by it; you know I think you're the best doctor in the world, and I love Ailin! It's just that those interns, or whatever they are down in the clinic, just can't seem to understand what I'm telling them about my back and my neck (pain); maybe they [referring to the foreign medical graduates] don't speak English well enough; they make me wait and wait, and it takes forever for them to order tests; I guess I'm just mad." The therapist then asked the rest of the group if anyone had had similar experiences in the clinic. A few of the other members agreed that they were frustrated by the long waits and test delays in the clinic, but no one shared the woman's feelings that the residents were not understanding them. The therapist then pressed the Irish-English-Scottish American woman, "You're angry at the Asian residents in the clinic because you feel they are not taking you seriously, and it comes out in a reference to 'Orientals not being good-looking.' I wonder if you're somehow feeling angry at me or are thinking I'm not listening to you." The woman replied, "Well, I guess maybe I don't like it that you're ending the group so soon."

The Asian therapist's technique of defusing the tension caused by the racially offensive comment was to use humor—not to make a joke or minimize the impact of the comment, but to point out how the remark was aimed at putting some distance between the member and herself. The therapist knew of the member's strong alliance with her in the treatment and the positive regard of the member toward her. She also knew that the Asian member was the only group member whom the Irish-English-Scottish American woman called and talked to outside of the group, and that there were strong positive feelings between them. Therefore, the therapist believed that the prejudiced remark about "Oriental doctors" was actually a barb at her, conveying a message that she felt an empathetic break. This issue could then be worked on prior to the end of the group.

Conclusion

The following modifications of technique have been found to be helpful in multiethnic, interpersonal group psychotherapy:

1. Encourage the explanation and exploration of ethnically derived values in order to help the members understand the interpersonal behavior that is the result of these values.
2. Help the members observe and understand nonverbal and symbolic forms of communication. Norms of self-expression will vary.
3. Explore the dynamics underlying the cultural transferences arising from group members, and examine cultural countertransferences occurring within the therapist(s).
4. Help the members examine their ethnic or racial prejudices in a safe environment that can contain the strong affects that arise.

Group psychotherapy with members of different ethnic groups is quite workable and may have some unique benefits. It creates a social microcosm in which members may safely try out new ways of relating, less restricted by their customary ethnic and cultural boundaries and social circles (Van der

Linden 1990). At times, a member will feel a freedom from his or her usual norms of communication, encouraged by others in the group to try something different.

The multiethnic therapy group is an environment in which one's differences are understood, and acceptance is gained on the basis of not only universally shared experiences but also particular experiences of ethnicity. That is, members with more symbolic and nonverbal modes of communication are accepted and understood as important, contributing members of the group, just as are the more direct and verbally expressive members. Experiences of being discriminated against because of race play a part in shaping one's relationships. The healing experience of being understood and helped in a group of people of different ethnicities, with diverse cultural values, may help one make desired changes in relationships.

References

Chen CC: Experiences with group psychotherapy in Taiwan. Int J Group Psychother 22:210–227, 1972

Chen CP: Group counseling in a different cultural context: several primary issues in dealing with Chinese clients. Group 19:45–55, 1995

Chu J, Sue S: Asian/Pacific-Americans and group practice. Social Work With Groups 7:23–35, 1984

Comas-Diaz L, Jacobsen FM: Ethnocultural identification in psychotherapy. Psychiatry 50:232–241, 1987

Davis LE: Essential components of group work with Black-Americans. Social Work With Groups 7:97–109, 1984

Delgado M: Hispanics and psychotherapeutic groups. Int J Group Psychother 33:507–520, 1983

Gehrie MJ: Culture as an internal representation. Psychiatry 42:165–170, 1979

Gilbert RK, Shiryaev E: Clinical psychology and psychotherapy in Russia: current status and future prospects. Journal of Humanistic Psychology 32:28–49, 1992

Hynes K, Werbin J: Group psychotherapy for Spanish-speaking women. Psychiatric Annals 7:52–63, 1977

Kinzie JD, Leung P, Bui A, et al: Cultural factors in group therapy with Southeast Asian refugees. Community Ment Health J 24:157–166, 1988

Knobel M: Significance and importance of the psychotherapist's personality and experience. Psychother Psychosom 53:58–63, 1990

Morsbach H: Aspects of nonverbal communication in Japan. J Nerv Ment Dis 157:262–277, 1973

Olarte SW, Masnik R: Group therapy for disadvantaged Hispanic outpatients. Hospital and Community Psychiatry 36:1093–1097, 1985

Ponce D: The Filipinos, in People and Cultures of Hawaii: A Psycho-Cultural Profile. Edited by McDermott JF Jr, Tseng WS, Maretzki TW. Honolulu, University of Hawaii Press, 1980, pp 155–163

Ridley CR: Racism in counseling as an adversive behavioral process, in Counseling Across Cultures. Edited by Pedersen PB, Draguns JG, Lonner WJ, et al. Honolulu, University of Hawaii Press, 1989, pp 55–77

Sugiyama-Lebra T: Japanese Patterns of Behavior. Honolulu, University of Hawaii Press, 1976

Tamura T, Lau A: Connectedness vs separateness: applicability of family therapy to Japanese families. Fam Process 31:319–340, 1992

Ticho GR: Cultural aspects of transference and countertransference. Bull Menninger Clin 35:313–326, 1971

Tsui P, Schultz GL: Failure of rapport: why psychotherapeutic engagement fails in the treatment of Asian clients. Am J Orthopsychiatry 55:561–569, 1985

Tsui P, Schultz GL: Ethnic factors in group process: cultural dynamics in multi-ethnic therapy groups. Am J Orthopsychiatry 58:136–142, 1988

Tylim I: Group psychotherapy with Hispanic patients: the psychodynamics of idealization. Int J Group Psychother 32:339–350, 1982

Van der Linden P: Anything valuable is vulnerable: individual values in therapeutic communities. International Journal of Therapeutic Communities 11:43–51, 1990

Vasquez MJT, Han AY: Group interventions and treatment with ethnic minorities, in Psychological Interventions and Cultural Diversity. Edited by Aponte JF, Rivers RY, Wohl J. Boston, MA, Allyn & Bacon, 1995, pp 109–127

Warriner CC: Planning and leading transcultural groups, in Transcultural Counseling: Needs, Programs and Techniques. Edited by Walz GR, Benjamin L. New York, Human Sciences Press, 1978, pp 127–152

White JC: The impact of race and ethnicity on transference and countertransference in combined individual/group therapy. Group 18:89–99, 1994

Wolman C: Group therapy in two languages, English and Navajo. Am J Psychother 24:677–685, 1970

Yamaguchi T: Group psychotherapy in Japan today. Int J Group Psychother 36:567–578, 1986

PART 6

Integration and Conclusions

CHAPTER 17

Integration and Conclusions

Wen-Shing Tseng, M.D.
Jon Streltzer, M.D.

Relevance of Culture to Psychotherapy

The influence of culture on psychotherapy has usually been viewed from a practical or technical perspective, but it is also extremely relevant when viewed from philosophical and theoretical perspectives. From a *philosophical* perspective, culture determines an individual's basic view of and attitude toward human beings, society, and the meaning of life, and thus will have an obvious impact on the patient in his or her search for improvement. When differences in cultural background exist between patient and therapist, there may also be differences in general philosophy and values. The psychotherapist needs to be aware of these differences, particularly when there is a need to help the patient evaluate the meaning of life, the implications of solving problems in life, and the direction the patient undertakes in life.

Culture certainly influences the *theoretical* basis for psychotherapy. Theories of psychology, including Freudian, Jungian, learning theory, ego psychology, and numerous others, are important, but more and more therapists consider themselves "eclectic," that is, choosing a therapeutic approach that will best fit the patient. The patient's cultural background and values help determine this fit.

In a related manner, theories explaining useful concepts, such as self, ego boundaries, personality, development, and defense mechanisms, may need cultural modifications when applied to different peoples. For the most part, these and related psychoanalytic concepts have been derived historically from clinical work with European and Euro-American patients. Such concepts have not been sufficiently tested with and revised for patients of other cultures. For instance, the boundary between self and others is less distinctly defined and more permeable within societies that encourage and foster interdependent relationships with family and others. Although the concept of personality development is universal, the pace of development and the major themes emphasized at each stage are subject to societal influence (e.g., the stage for autonomy is much delayed, and the theme of independence is less emphasized in many cultures). The concept of defense mechanism is universally applicable, yet there is room for cultural revision, particularly with regard to the hierarchy of "maturity" of defense mechanisms. Theoretical issues such as these await cross-cultural modification and consequent application to the practice of psychotherapy with patients of different cultures.

At another stratum, it is well recognized that culture often influences *technical* issues, including the mode and manner of therapy and various clinical issues within the therapy. The modern therapist has many choices: individual, couples, family, or group; interpersonal; cognitive-behavioral; supportive; crisis-oriented; passive versus directive; and so forth. In addition to the choice of type of therapy, specific areas such as the therapist-patient relationship, assessment of pathology, meaning of interpretations and other communications, role of the family, and goals, often are influenced by cultural factors, which may be readily apparent or quite subtle.

Although this book has emphasized a focus on culture in treating different ethnic groups, we do not mean to limit the scope that way. The same principles apply to subcultures within a larger society, and in a sense each individual has his or her own unique culture. Cultural principles also apply to the psychotherapy of special populations, such as patients of minority backgrounds (Aponte et al. 1995), different social classes (Foster et al. 1996), different sexual orientations (Greene 1997), or with physical handicaps. Such patients may be so different from the therapist in their life experiences and views of the world that empathy across this barrier of "difference" is needed.

Universality Versus Cultural Specificity

Psychopathology has varying degrees of universal elements and cultural influences (Tseng and Streltzer 1997), and, likewise, psychotherapy incorporates many nonspecific universal healing elements, such as the exercise of a powerful, authoritative figure and mobilization of resource persons, allowing emotional ventilation, channeling of inhibited desires, and cultivation of hope (Frank 1961; Torrey 1986). These universal elements are a critical part of any psychotherapy, no matter how prominent cultural elements seem to be.

More often than not, cultural elements are rather subtle and are most valuable in the way that they can be incorporated to help maximize the universal healing powers of psychotherapy. For example, the decision to uncover or to suppress issues of emotional consequence may be determined by the cultural influences on the patient's individual psychology. The correct decision is the one that allows the universal therapeutic mechanisms to be the most effective, and this is usually the one that is most consonant with the patient's culture.

Sociocultural Background of the Patient and Family

To conduct psychotherapy in a culturally relevant way, the therapist must pay attention to the sociocultural context within which the therapy is going to take place. The therapist need not be a cultural anthropologist, but, from a practical point of view, he or she needs to become an expert in the specific cultural background of the patient being treated. This is particularly true when the patient belongs to a culture that diverges from that of the therapist.

Useful areas to know include the patient's values, beliefs, customs, rituals, and common patterns of behavior, and how these match or diverge from the norms of the patient's culture. To determine such, it helps to learn about the sociocultural background in which the patient grew up: the social structure, family system, political ideology, and economic conditions; the medical system itself; the prominence of folk healing; the history of medicine and psychiatry; and the population's general understanding and attitude toward mental illness and emotional problems. These factors may influence the direction of psychotherapy in very practical ways.

For patients of minority ethnicity, it is important to recognize how their group is perceived by the larger society. What are the stereotypes? Has the group been subject to discrimination and prejudice? If these issues are important, but missed or ignored by the therapist, then empathy will be difficult, if not impossible, to achieve.

Knowledge of the family system is often particularly valuable. Although the importance of family is universal, there are wide cultural variations in the role of men versus women, the freedom to develop relationships outside the family, child-rearing practices, and so forth (Tseng and Hsu 1991).

Levels of Cultural Influence on Psychotherapy

Motivation for Therapy

Not every person is "psychologically minded" in the contemporary mental health sense and has a clear idea about the nature and process of psychotherapy. The level of psychological mindedness may vary generally from society to society, as well as from individual to individual, on the basis of common attitudes toward mental illness or emotional problems, overall medical knowledge and sophistication, general appreciation of the process of introspection, and acceptance of help from an outside "expert." The patient's cultural background may provide clues that enable the therapist to maximize the patient's motivation for therapy. For example, the therapist may choose to stimulate the patient's curiosity, exert direct authority, or enlist family support. Such approaches are more likely to be necessary at the beginning of treatment when the patient is a new immigrant or a member of a minority group.

The Presenting Problem

The patient's presenting problem usually leads the direction of the therapy—at least in the initial stage. As a part of the illness behavior, the patient's style of reporting suffering will be shaped by cultural factors. How a person chooses a topic or focuses the presentation of clinical problems is subject to individual need and understanding of the health system, but is also very much influenced by the culturally patterned style of problem presentation. The patient's explanations and beliefs about problems may cover a broad spectrum of the supernatural, natural, biophysical, medical, and psychological. The nature of the problems may be presented as somatic, psychological, or a combination of the two. The patient's problem presentation needs to be understood dynamically within the context of the patient's cultural background (Tseng 1975).

Goals of Therapy

The goals of psychotherapy may be influenced by cultural factors. The concept of "normality" may be defined in different ways, such as by statistical means; on the basis of expert opinions or functional capabilities; and from sociocultural perspectives (Offer and Sabshin 1975). The definition of "healthy," "mature," and "adaptive" may be very different, depending on the value system held by a group of people in a particular cultural setting. There- fore, the therapist needs to negotiate the purpose of the therapy and its ex- pected benefits, and perhaps even some of the mechanics of the therapy, taking into consideration the sociocultural environment and perspective of the patient.

Therapist-Patient Relationship

The relationship established between the therapist and the patient will often determine the success of the psychotherapy. While the type of therapy (e.g., dynamic, supportive, cognitive-behavioral, brief, long-term) has major impli- cations for this relationship, cultural considerations may also have powerful effects. For example, there may be cultural expectations that the therapist should take an authoritative, active, and giving role in relating to the patient; or, in contrast, the therapist may be expected to relate to the patient on a rel- atively equal basis, without interfering with the patient's autonomy and in- dependence.

The quality of the therapist-patient relationship becomes an obvious is- sue that is critical in therapy when there is a cultural gap. When the therapist and patient have different ethnic/cultural backgrounds, particularly involv- ing majority-minority differences, the relationship must be examined care- fully, not only from the beginning but throughout the course of therapy. Ignoring relationship issues under these circumstances renders the therapy highly problematic.

Ethnic Matching of Therapist and Patient

The pros and cons of matching the ethnic/cultural backgrounds of therapist and patient have been a matter of debate for cultural psychotherapists for some time (Comas-Diaz 1988; Griffith 1977; Sundberg and Sue 1989; Yama- moto et al. 1993). Matching the ethnic or racial background may seem de- sirable in that cultural empathy might be maximized with less chance of misunderstanding, but such matching is not always feasible. Furthermore, it can be advantageous for a therapist to be of a different cultural background. The patient may feel less likely to "lose face" to an outsider, who may be more readily accepted as nonjudgmental. The therapist may also plead igno- rance of the patient's cultural background, thus facilitating more thorough explanations, which, in turn, lead to greater understanding of, and connec- tion with, the individual patient.

Racial/Ethnic Transference and Countertransference

The therapeutic relationship involves ordinary and realistic aspects, as well as specific individual transference and countertransference elements. When there is a cultural gap between therapist and patient, one may consider additional racial, ethnic, or cultural aspects of the transference and countertransference. Culture is an abstract concept, whose existence may be barely recognized if one has not developed a specific interest in or sensitivity to it. Yet race and ethnicity are concrete and obvious. Thus, although transference or countertransference is often related to ethnicity or race, it is seldom recognized and identified as cultural in nature. Racial or ethnic-derived transference and countertransference, like individual-specific transference and countertransference, can be manifested in various ways, profoundly influencing the process of therapy. Thus, these elements need attending to from the very beginning of therapy, particularly if prejudicial stereotypes are involved.

Impact of Therapist's Value System

The therapist is likely to be highly educated, to be financially secure, to have high social status, and to see life as fulfilling and rewarding of good effort. The therapist is likely to believe that his or her value system is a healthy and functional one and, therefore, ideal for the patient too. Yet, from a cultural perspective, the therapist's values are not necessarily useful to the patient, or even relevant to the patient's circumstances and cultural background. A clinician needs to be aware of the possible irrelevance of his or her personal values and to constantly assess and regulate the therapy to maintain its cultural appropriateness.

Several issues are particularly vulnerable to culturally driven values. For example, the therapist may value autonomy, independence, and individual achievement in contrast to the patient of non-Western background, who values interdependence and fitting in with the group (Doi 1973). A Western therapist may perceive dependent behavior as pathological, whereas an Asian therapist may consider the same behavior as perfectly normal. The therapist may have values and expectations different from those of the patient regarding the status of women, which varies widely in different cultures. Culture is also a strong determinant of the relative acceptance of passive versus aggressive behavior. Other good examples are the attitude and behavioral expectations of the child toward the parent and, in a related fashion, the attitude toward authority in general. These cultural values often have profound implications for the doctor-patient relationship.

Language and Communication Style

If the patient and the therapist do not share a common language, an interpreter needs to be used to provide an alternative mode of communication. Since the nature of psychotherapy is communication, conducting it indirectly through a third party is burdensome and complicates the process of therapy. The nature of the interpretation has significant implications for the therapy. The interpreter may provide word-to-word translation or a summary translation, or may offer additional opinions about what the patient really means, or even what the therapist should be saying! Furthermore, many concepts and feeling states cannot easily be comprehended and translated from one language to another. The therapist must recognize that the translation may be an equivalence or an approximation. Empathy is more difficult, and the therapeutic value of emotional catharsis will be limited when attempted indirectly or through a secondary language. Even when therapist and patient communicate in the same language, special attention must be given to the nature of the communication that takes place, including the content, level of sophistication, and focus of communication. This is particularly true when a therapist is going to provide explanations, interpretations, or suggestions for the patient or the patient's family. The same words may have different symbolic meanings in different cultural contexts.

General Issues in Psychotherapy

Family Participation in Therapy

Although family therapists have traditionally been strong advocates for their treatment techniques, many clinicians have believed that individual therapy is more definitive for most patients. Family sessions can be invaluable, however, in treating patients from other ethnic groups, particularly minorities or cultural groups that stress the importance of family ties in their social relationships. Such sessions are especially helpful in the early stages of therapy or if the treatment seems to get stuck. Working with family members assists the therapist in learning about the culture of the patient. This, in turn, helps the therapist to understand the nature of the individual problems and the importance of family relations to the genesis of the problems and their solution. Working with family members also may help the therapist to predict the effects of attempted therapeutic interventions.

Prescription of Medication

With the great advances in psychopharmacology, it has become commonplace for a patient to receive medication while undergoing psychotherapy. In some settings, it is rare for the patient *not* to receive medication. Prescribing medication for patients is not purely a biological-medical matter, but involves significant psychological issues as well, including cultural meanings for giving and receiving medication. Medication is strongly associated with the image of a healer. The interaction between doctor and patient around medication issues can be therapeutic, particularly if such use is harmonious with cultural beliefs. In addition, a focus on medication may allow a face-saving way of avoiding direct exposure of emotional issues, which may then be reached indirectly.

Culturally Specific Issues in Therapy

Ethnic/Cultural Identity Issues

Ethnic identity and *cultural identity* are rather abstract terms that are often difficult to grasp. Nevertheless, many patients, particularly those with low self-esteem, are confused about their cultural identity, or they devalue it. In a subtle way, such confusion or devaluation can cause much suffering over a lifetime. If the therapist has the same cultural background as the patient, then a positive personal identification with the therapist can be very therapeutic in and of itself. If the therapist is from a different cultural background, then the therapist's high valuation of the patient's culture can be equally therapeutic (Comas-Diaz and Jacobsen 1987).

Cohort or generation issues may also influence cultural identity. The patient may have been raised in a culture that is now having dramatic changes in its younger generations. In a somewhat similar fashion, acculturation issues can lead to identity conflicts. For patients of mixed ethnicity, conflicts associated with identity may be particularly problematic. The therapist may need to communicate appreciation for both (several) cultures or for the specialness of the patient.

Therapy With Intercultural Couples, Families, and Groups

The treatment of couples, families, or groups whose members have racial, ethnic, or cultural differences becomes a special challenge for the therapist. There may be cultural differences in patterns of communication, as well as expectations of duties, obligations, commitment or relatedness to others, and collective identification. In these situations, ethnic or cultural identity issues often become very explicit and need to be dealt with actively and skillfully. The clinician acts not only as a psychotherapist but also as a culture broker, in that he or she must find ways to interpret meanings and values that each involved party can accept, thus fostering communication and allowing progress toward common therapeutic goals.

Unusual and Supernatural Cultural Beliefs

The contemporary psychotherapist may be confronted by a patient who has unusual cultural beliefs, such as a belief in the supernatural. This can be paralyzing to the therapist who has been educated in rational scientific thinking. For instance, a patient may complain that she is cursed for breaking a taboo. Another patient may obsess about the appearance of his deceased mother's spirit in his dream, believing this means she was not properly worshipped by her children after her death. An Asian patient may complain that the level of *chi* is declining in his body (*chi* refers to an abstract but fundamental force that exists within the body to regulate function). This patient's complaint is similar to the complaint of a Hispanic patient that he has lost his soul or spirit. For Westerners, many beliefs of a supernatural nature are often accepted comfortably in the context of religion; however, culturally related supernatural beliefs that do not fit in with Western religious thought tend to be regarded as superstitions.

The culture-oriented therapist must be flexible in dealing with unusual or supernatural cultural beliefs. He or she may need to learn about the beliefs from the patient, or by doing outside research, in order to put the issue in the proper context. Hidden psychological conflicts amenable to therapy may emerge. The unusual beliefs may also have symbolic or metaphoric meanings and may culturally serve a social function.

Somatization of Psychological Problems

Cartesian dualism permeates Western thinking about mind and body, viewing them as characteristically distinct things. This philosophical view has specific ramifications in Western medical practice, in which bodily complaints are expected to be qualitatively different from psychological complaints, leading to different treatment approaches. Eastern thinking tends to see harmony, or connectedness, in all things, a holistic point of view. Mind and body are not qualitatively different from this perspective, but more like different ways of looking at the whole person. From the Western perspective, Asian patients are thought to often somatize psychological problems, but from a non-Western perspective it appears that Western cultures are likely to psychologize problems (Kirmayer 1989).

When the non-Western patient presents somatic complaints in psychotherapy, this does not necessarily imply resistance to psychological issues.

Rather, it may be very useful to express interest in and concern over such complaints, at least initially, and to gradually allow personal conflicts to be addressed. Concern over somatic complaints can symbolically validate the healer-patient relationship. On the other hand, it is important for the therapist not to get stuck in an exclusive focus on the somatic complaints, because then he or she will be unable to demonstrate healing power.

Qualities Necessary for Culturally Competent Psychotherapy

A clinically competent psychotherapist is expected to be knowledgeable about theories of human behavior and psychopathology. The therapist is expected to be skilled at applying this knowledge to clinical assessment and the choice of psychotherapeutic technique. The therapist should be caring, sensitive, and experienced in clinical work.

Culturally competent psychotherapy requires additional qualities. The therapist must be able to put the patient's situation in a cultural context. Psychotherapeutic interventions must be chosen on the basis of cultural considerations, not just a narrow view of psychopathology. The therapist may need to help the patient with aspects of cultural adjustment. These interventions may include helping the ethnic minority patient to maintain a healthy ethnic identity and, at the same time, adjust to the society of the majority; supporting the immigrant to maintain a core cultural identity while acculturating into the host society; or resolving conflict in a family with a severe generation gap problem due to rapid sociocultural changes. The culturally competent therapist may be called on to maintain, change, balance, or integrate multiple subcultural systems for the individual of mixed ethnicity, the couple with different cultural backgrounds, or the family that consists of several ethnicities. These skills require special qualities: cultural sensitivity, cultural knowledge, cultural empathy, and cultural insight.

Cultural Sensitivity

Cultural sensitivity refers to a clinical quality of being open and sensitive to the dimension of culture in human behavior and of having an appreciation of the different attitudes, beliefs, and perspectives that are held by people of different social, political, economic, ethnic, and religious groups. Cultural sensitivity requires a determination to avoid being ethnocentric and an eagerness to learn, understand, and accept another's culture, with the knowledge that potential differences exist. It also refers to the ability to appreciate that not only are "they" different from me, but "I" am different from them, so that the therapist is aware of his or her own value system and will constantly examine how his or her attitudes, beliefs, and values may intrude on the therapy and affect the patient.

Cultural Knowledge

Culturally competent therapy requires *knowledge* about the patient's cultural background. This knowledge need not be comprehensive and in depth, but it should cover basic areas and then be developed specifically to fit the individual patient. Such knowledge should be put in the context of a general knowledge of cultural influences on psychopathology (Tseng and Streltzer 1997). On occasion, anthropological reading, or consultation with a medical anthropologist or other cultural informant, may be helpful, in a general way, to understand the patient's culture. More often, the patient's family or friends may be a good resource for knowledge of the patient's culture—as long as the therapist is careful to distinguish among ideal, practical, or stereotyped cultural information. Most often, however, the most useful and practical source of information is the patient himself or herself, who is likely to appreciate the attention and interest of the therapist. The patient not only can teach the therapist about his or her culture but also can reveal the significance of cultural beliefs and values to the issues being treated.

Cultural Empathy

If the therapist is sensitive to cultural issues and develops knowledge about the patient's culture, then he or she will have the potential for *cultural empathy*. Such empathy involves going beyond awareness of what one might feel being in the patient's situation. It requires an understanding of the emotional reactions of the patient because of an ability to view the situation *from the patient's cultural perspective*. Otherwise, a gap in understanding will remain, and the therapist will be unable to participate in the emotional experience of the patient. Cultural empathy is an important ability that may well determine the quality of the psychotherapy.

Cultural Insight

Finally, *cultural insight* is needed when the psychotherapeutic process may directly impinge on important cultural issues. Culturally determined norms, values, and goals may need to be challenged and adjusted in order to treat problems or resolve conflicts. Culturally sanctioned coping mechanisms may need reinforcement, or, if ineffective, they may need to be confronted. Alternatives to culturally defined solutions may need to be proposed. Such psychotherapeutic processes can change culturally influenced issues, but they must do so in culturally appropriate ways. Psychotherapy involves the interaction of two value systems—the patient's and the therapist's—providing opportunities for exposure, exchange, and incorporation of differing cultural elements (Tseng and Hsu 1979). Cultural insight allows regulation of this interaction and of the overall therapeutic process in a culturally competent manner.

Conclusion

The practice of psychotherapy is a complex matter. The process is determined by various factors, including the nature of the psychological problems faced by the patient, the character strengths of the patient, the patient's usual coping mechanisms, the motivation for therapy, the therapist-patient relationship, the therapist's treatment strategies and techniques, the stage of treatment and ongoing developments, the goals of therapy, and any potential socioeconomic restrictions affecting the length or type of treatment.

Beyond these general clinical and social factors, cultural issues may powerfully influence the process and outcome of psychotherapy and, therefore, deserve special attention. Cultural considerations are clearly important when the patient's cultural background differs from that of the therapist or when culture-specific problems or syndromes are being treated. This is usually the case when the patient belongs to a special population group, such as immigrants or minorities, including those defined by race, ethnicity, social status, sexual preference, or physical handicap.

However, we also believe that the principles of cultural psychotherapy are more broadly applicable and, in fact, apply to *every* patient for whom psychotherapy is appropriate. This includes patients of majority ethnicity and of long-standing geographical affiliation. Every patient has a unique personality, family constellation, and sociocultural circumstance that guides his or her way of thinking, feeling, and behaving. Since every individual is unique, he or she cannot be stereotyped with regard to attitudes, beliefs, and values. Thus, a true cultural understanding of any given patient will be unique to that patient. An understanding of the patient's broader cultural background can only be an approximation, helping the therapist toward an appreciation of the patient's particular individuality. Therefore, cultural considerations are necessary in treating any patient, even when the patient shares the same ethnic and broader cultural background with the therapist. There will always be differences between patient and therapist with regard to educational and occupational history, faith, socioeconomic level, family values, life experiences, and so forth.

Also, we believe that *every* therapist—whether minority or majority, whatever the ethnicity or cultural background—needs to constantly examine and manage his or her own cultural beliefs, attitudes, and, particularly, values when conducting psychotherapy. The therapist's culturally based values can overtly or tacitly influence both the content and the process of psychotherapy.

In conclusion, cultural factors influence, and are involved in, psychotherapy in many ways. Interest in the patient's culture, and attention to the various implications of culture during the therapeutic process, will enhance the relevance and success of psychotherapy.

References

Aponte JF, Rivers RY, Wohl J (eds): Psychological Interventions and Cultural Diversity. Boston, Allyn & Bacon, 1995

Comas-Diaz L: Cross-cultural mental health treatment, in Clinical Guidelines in Cross-Cultural Mental Health. Edited by Comas-Diaz L, Griffith EEH. New York, Wiley, 1988

Comas-Diaz L, Jacobsen FM: Ethnocultural identification in psychotherapy. Psychiatry 50:232–241, 1987

Doi T: The Anatomy of Dependence: The Key Analysis of Japanese Behavior. Tokyo, Kodansha International, 1973

Foster RMP, Moskowitz M, Javier RA (eds): Reaching Across Boundaries of Culture and Class: Widening the Scope of Psychotherapy. Northvale, NJ, Jason Aronson, 1996

Frank JD: Persuasion and Healing: A Comparative Study of Psychotherapy. New York, Schocken, 1961

Greene B (ed): Ethnic and Cultural Diversity Among Lesbians and Gay Men. Thousand Oaks, CA, Sage, 1997

Griffith MS: The influence of race on the psychotherapeutic relationship. Psychiatry 40:27–40, 1977

Kirmayer LJ: Psychotherapy and the cultural concept of the person. Sante, Culture, Health 6:241–270, 1989

Offer D, Sabshin M: Normality, in Comprehensive Textbook of Psychiatry/II, 2nd Edition, Vol 1. Edited by Freedman AM, Kaplan HI, Sadock BJ. Baltimore, MD, Williams & Wilkins, 1975, pp 459–464

Sundberg ND, Sue D: Research and research hypotheses about effectiveness in intercultural counseling, in Counseling Across Cultures, 3rd Edition. Edited by Pedersen PB, Draguns JG, Lonner WJ, et al. Honolulu, University of Hawaii Press, 1989, pp 335–370

Torrey EF: Witchdoctors and Psychiatrists: The Common Roots of Psychotherapy and Its Future. New York, Harper & Row, 1986

Tseng WS: The nature of somatic complaints among psychiatric patients: the Chinese case. Compr Psychiatry 16:237–245, 1975

Tseng WS, Hsu J: Culture and psychotherapy, in Perspectives on Cross-Cultural Psychology. Edited by Marsella AJ, Tharp RG, Ciborowski TJ. New York, Academic Press, 1979, pp 333–345

Tseng WS, Hsu J: Culture and Family: Problems and Therapy. New York, Haworth Press, 1991

Tseng WS, Streltzer J (eds): Culture and Psychopathology: A Guide to Clinical Assessment. New York, Brunner/Mazel, 1997

Yamamoto J, Silva JA, Justice LR, et al: Cross-cultural psychotherapy, in Culture, Ethnicity, and Mental Illness. Edited by Gaw AC. Washington, DC, American Psychiatric Press, 1993, pp 101–124

Index